NEUROSURGERY PRACTICE QUESTIONS AND ANSWERS

Second Edition

NEUROSURGERY PRACTICE QUESTIONS AND ANSWERS

Second Edition

Mark R. Shaya, MD, FACS
Founder and President
Neurosurgical Institute of Florida
Miami, Florida

Cristian Gragnaniello, MD, PhD, MSurg, MAdvSurg, FICS
Surgical Director
Harvey H. Ammerman Microsurgical Laboratory
Department of Neurosurgery
George Washington University
Washington, DC

Remi Nader, MD, CM, FRCS(C), FAANS, FACS
Founder and President
Texas Center for Neurosciences
Houston, Texas

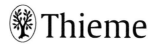

Executive Editor: Timothy Y. Hiscock
Managing Editor: Sarah Landis
Director, Editorial Services: Mary Jo Casey
Assistant Managing Editor: Nikole Connors
Production Editor: Sean Woznicki
International Production Director: Andreas Schabert
Vice President, Editorial and E-Product Development:
  Vera Spillner
International Marketing Director: Fiona Henderson
International Sales Director: Louisa Turrell
Director of Sales, North America: Mike Roseman
Senior Vice President and Chief Operating Officer:
Sarah Vanderbilt
President: Brian D. Scanlan

Library of Congress Cataloging-in-Publication Data

Names: Shaya, Mark, author. | Gragnaniello, Cristian, author.
  | Nader, Remi, author.
Title: Neurosurgery practice questions and answers /
  Mark R. Shaya, Cristian Gragnaniello, Remi Nader.
Description: 2nd edition. | New York : Thieme, [2016]
Identifiers: LCCN 2016023304 | ISBN 9781626233478
Subjects: | MESH: Neurosurgical Procedures | Nervous
  System Diseases--surgery | Neurosurgery--methods |
  Examination Questions
Classification: LCC RC356 | NLM WL 18.2 | DDC 616.80076--
  dc23 LC record available at https://lccn.loc.gov/2016023304

© 2016 Thieme Medical Publishers, Inc.

Thieme Publishers New York
333 Seventh Avenue, New York, NY 10001 USA
+1 800 782 3488, customerservice@thieme.com

Thieme Publishers Stuttgart
Rüdigerstrasse 14, 70469 Stuttgart, Germany
+49 [0]711 8931 421, customerservice@thieme.de

Thieme Publishers Delhi
A-12, Second Floor, Sector-2, Noida-201301
Uttar Pradesh, India
+91 120 45 566 00, customerservice@thieme.in

Thieme Publishers Rio de Janeiro, Thieme Publicações
  Ltda.
Edifício Rodolpho de Paoli, 25º andar
Av. Nilo Peçanha, 50 – Sala 2508,
Rio de Janeiro 20020-906 Brasil
+55 21 3172-2297 / +55 21 3172-1896

Cover design: Thieme Publishing Group
Typesetting by DiTech Process Solutions

Printed in the United States of America by
  Sheridan Press   5 4 3 2 1

ISBN 978-1-62623-347-8

Also available as an e-book:
eISBN 978-1-62623-364-5

Important note: Medicine is an ever-changing science undergoing continual development. Research and clinical experience are continually expanding our knowledge, in particular our knowledge of proper treatment and drug therapy. Insofar as this book mentions any dosage or application, readers may rest assured that the authors, editors, and publishers have made every effort to ensure that such references are in accordance with **the state of knowledge at the time of production of the book.**

Nevertheless, this does not involve, imply, or express any guarantee or responsibility on the part of the publishers in respect to any dosage instructions and forms of applications stated in the book. **Every user is requested to examine carefully** the manufacturers' leaflets accompanying each drug and to check, if necessary in consultation with a physician or specialist, whether the dosage schedules mentioned therein or the contraindications stated by the manufacturers differ from the statements made in the present book. Such examination is particularly important with drugs that are either rarely used or have been newly released on the market. Every dosage schedule or every form of application used is entirely at the user's own risk and responsibility. The authors and publishers request every user to report to the publishers any discrepancies or inaccuracies noticed. If errors in this work are found after publication, errata will be posted at www.thieme.com on the product description page.

Some of the product names, patents, and registered designs referred to in this book are in fact registered trademarks or proprietary names even though specific reference to this fact is not always made in the text. Therefore, the appearance of a name without designation as proprietary is not to be construed as a representation by the publisher that it is in the public domain.

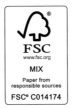

Dedicated to those neurosurgeons without the titles of academia or positions in societies, but oftentimes with the most skill, wisdom, and experience: the private practice neurosurgeon.

Content

Foreword

Dr. Mark Shaya, Dr. Remi Nader, and Dr. Cristian Gragnaniello have produced a beautiful, balanced and thorough tome that addresses a growing need in neurosurgery. This second edition of *Neurosurgery Practice Questions and Answers* is a valuable tool for continuing education and, more importantly, a tool for board and maintenance of certification examination preparation. They present over 800 prototypical board examination questions and answers featuring in-depth explanations for answers.

With the relentless and endless perpetual increase in the body of neurosurgical knowledge, neurosurgeons are faced with incredible educational difficulties. This book will most certainly serve as a unique and valid mechanism to help address this challenge.

Practicing neurosurgeons can refer to this book as a simple refresher. It most certainly will be extraordinarily useful as a preparation tool for maintenance of certification examinations. Residents in training can similarly use this book as a tool for knowledge acquisition and for board preparation. This book can also effectively serve as a platform for the pursuit of knowledge; the more challenging questions in the book will help the reader to identify knowledge gaps where further study is needed.

The question topics are diverse and cover the entire field of neurosurgery, including all sub-disciplines. In addition, the questions blanket the associated basic science fields—these include pharmacology, physiology, anatomy, and pathology. Finally, imaging and neurology questions broaden the scope of the book even further, thus making it truly relevant to board and maintenance of certification examination preparation

In summary, this book represents an inexpensive and very valuable tool for neurosurgery education. It belongs on the shelf of every neurosurgeon and neurosurgery trainee.

Edward Benzel, MD
Chairman, Department of Neurosurgery
Neurological Institute, Cleveland Clinic
Cleveland, Ohio

Preface

I am glad to present to you this second edition of *Neurosurgery Practice Questions and Answers*. This book project originally started in about 2003 when I was a resident. It was a pure labor of love and also a good reason to collaborate with neurosurgery friends and colleagues. Working on this second edition, I am amazed by how far neurosurgery has come in just the past decade. Medications, treatments, and diagnostic studies which were novel and state of the art in the first edition of this book are now routine in this second edition. One can only imagine about the future and wonder what will happen to our field in another ten years.

Neurosurgery is changing not only scientifically but also clinically and administratively. We are entering an era of high regulation, cost-sensitive care, maintenance of certification, and computerized patient documentation. While these things are meant to improve the quality of care, they can at times diminish the art of medicine and surgery. I remember being a student and witnessing a wonderful hand-written neurosurgical consultation by an attending neurosurgeon; beautifully hand-drawn sketches in the margins depicted the patient's symptoms with the surgeon's thoughts numbered at the bottom of the page as a differential diagnosis. I believe this is how most neurosurgeons think when solving a surgical problem. But such neurosurgical problem solving is now being replaced with computerized template notes which, although thorough, do not fully capture a complex neurosurgical situation and the subtle intangibles of our patients. Moreover, the controversial maintenance of certification process takes precious time away from our patients; it is still in a flux and there is significant pressure from the neurosurgical community to lessen its current impact on their practices. All of these are obstacles not only for the neurosurgeon finishing residency but also for the established neurosurgeon both in an academic or private setting. We must not let these matters lessen our motivation to use our surgical instincts nor restrict our creative abilities, since it is with our creativity and imagination that progress in neurosurgery usually originates.

I would like to thank Remi Nader and Cristian Gragnaniello for their assistance with this second edition; also, thanks to Gauri Wable and Sohum Desai for their contributions to this book. I sincerely hope that this work will assist in your examination preparation no matter what level you are preparing for.

Mark R. Shaya, MD, FACS
Founder and President
Neurosurgical Institute of Florida
Miami, Florida

Questions

1. Regarding the pathophysiology of myasthenia gravis, what is/are the possible mechanisms by which acetylcholine receptor antibodies interfere with neuromuscular transmission?
   A. Binding to the acetylcholine receptor and blocking the binding of acetylcholine
   B. Cross-linking acetylcholine receptors, thereby increasing their rate of internalization
   C. Binding of complement resulting in destruction of the muscle end plate
   D. All of the above
   E. None of the above

2. All of the following statements are correct regarding the medial lemniscus EXCEPT:
   A. Near the sensory decussation, its blood supply comes from the anterior spinal artery.
   B. The medial lemniscus can be found in close proximity to the anterolateral tract in the medulla. Its somatotopy in the pons is such that leg fibers are lateral to arm fibers.
   C. The fibers of the medial lemniscus arise from the cuneate and gracile nuclei.
   D. Brainstem lesions involving medial lemniscus fibers usually include adjacent structures, resulting in motor and sensory losses.
   E. None of the above statements are correct.

3. All the following findings are associated with the abnormality seen on the scan shown here EXCEPT:

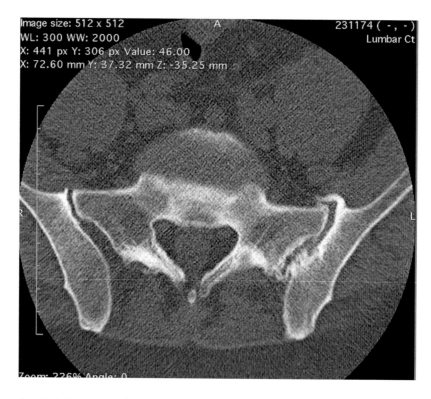

A. Ankylosing spondylitis
B. Positive FABER test
C. Positive thigh thrust
D. Pain upon internal rotation of the hip
E. Positive thigh compression text

4. Which of the following lines at the craniocervical junction extends from the basion to the opisthion?
A. McRae's line
B. McGregor's line
C. Chamberlain's line
D. Wackenheim's line
E. Anterior marginal line

5. The somatotopic arrangement in the ventral horn is such that the
A. flexors are dorsal to extensors and limbs are medial to trunk.
B. extensors are dorsal to flexors and limbs are medial to trunk.
C. flexors are dorsal to extensors and limbs are lateral to trunk.
D. extensors are dorsal to flexors and limbs are lateral to trunk.
E. None of the above

6. All of the following techniques may be used to aid in identifying the level of interest in a thoracic diskectomy procedure EXCEPT:
    A. Intraoperative lateral fluoroscopy with counting levels starting from the sacrum and moving rostral with midline needle localizers
    B. Intraoperative anteroposterior (AP) fluoroscopy with counting levels starting from the 12th rib and moving rostral with midline needle localizers
    C. Intraoperative AP fluoroscopy with counting levels starting from the first rib and moving caudal with midline needle localizers
    D. Neuronavigation with skin surface fiducial registration
    E. Neuronavigation with spinal bony landmark registration within the proximity of the level of interest

7. The MRI scan shown here represents an opportunistic infection in a 25-year-old man with acute myelogenous leukemia. All the following statements are true EXCEPT:

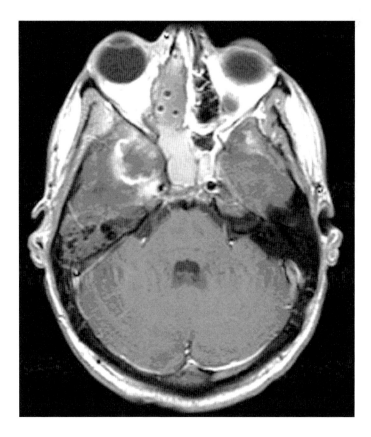

    A. Pathology reveals pleomorphic short and wide septate hyphae.
    B. It can be treated with Cancidas, voriconazole, and AmBisome.
    C. It causes hemorrhagic necrosis and ischemic strokes.
    D. The organism originates in the soil.
    E. It may be seen with an immunocompromised patient.

8.   Somatic motor efferents to the urethral sphincter are located in
   A.   intermediolateral cell columns of the sacral cord.
   B.   Onuf's nucleus.
   C.   Barrington's nucleus.
   D.   All of the above
   E.   None of the above

9.   Cerebral ischemia begins when cerebral perfusion pressure (CPP) falls below
   A.   100 mm Hg.
   B.   75 mm Hg.
   C.   50 mm Hg.
   D.   23 mm Hg.
   E.   8 mm Hg.

10.   Regarding the anatomy near the cavernous sinus, the borders of the clinoidal triangle are cranial nerves
   A.   I and II.
   B.   II and III.
   C.   III and IV.
   D.   IV and V.
   E.   None of the above

11.   Which of the following is FALSE regarding myasthenia gravis?
   A.   The first presentation is usually weakness of the extraocular muscles.
   B.   Weakness fluctuates and fatigues over the course of the day.
   C.   Speech may be hypernasal or hoarse in some patients.
   D.   It may present with a head drop.
   E.   Dysphagia is worst at breakfast and improves during the course of the day.

12.   All of the following are true of polymyositis EXCEPT:
   A.   It involves a symmetric weakness of proximal limb and trunk muscles.
   B.   Its onset is insidious.
   C.   Ocular muscles are usually spared.
   D.   Muscles are not tender to palpation.
   E.   Skin changes typically occur before muscle abnormalities.

13.   *Protein 14-3-3* is elevated in the CSF in which of the following conditions?
   A.   Creutzfeldt-Jakob disease
   B.   Demyelinating disease
   C.   Head trauma
   D.   Meningoencephalitis
   E.   All of the above

14. Which of the following statements is most accurate regarding the nerve supplying the teres minor muscle?
    A. It has a contribution from the lateral cord.
    B. It is an extension of the posterior cord.
    C. Ventral rami C8 and T1 are major contributors to this nerve.
    D. It is derived from the same cord as the musculocutaneous nerve.
    E. None of the above

15. The pterion is formed by the junction of the all of the following EXCEPT:
    A. Frontal bone
    B. Sphenoid bone
    C. Zygomatic bone
    D. Temporal bone
    E. Parietal bone

16. Which of the following is FALSE regarding the sonic hedgehog (SHH) gene?
    A. SHH has been found to have the critical roles in development of the limb and midline structures in the brain and spinal cord.
    B. Mutations in the human SHH gene, cause holoprosencephaly type 3 as a result of the loss of the ventral midline.
    C. The SHH transcription pathway has been linked to the formation of embryonic cerebellar tumors such as medulloblastoma.
    D. SHH has been shown to act as an axonal guidance cue: SHH attracts retinal ganglion cell axons at high concentrations and repels them at lower concentrations.
    E. SHH plays a critical role in the induction of the floor plate and diverse ventral cell types within the neural tube.

17. Regarding infection in a trauma patient with the X-ray shown here, the most common pathogen is

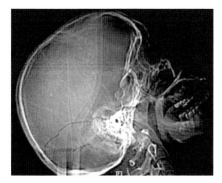

    A. *Staphylococcus aureus.*
    B. *Pseudomonas.*
    C. *Proteus.*
    D. *Streptococcus pneumoniae.*
    E. *Escherichia coli.*

18. Which of the following is incorrect regarding the zona incerta?
   A. It is a zone of gray matter between the thalamic and lenticular fasciculi.
   B. It is composed of cells that are continuous laterally with the thalamic reticular nucleus.
   C. Unlike the thalamic reticular nucleus, the neurons of this zone do not display immunoreactivity for the calcium binding protein calbindin D-28k.
   D. It receives corticofugal fibers from the precentral cortex.
   E. All of the above statements are correct.

19. All the following are potential contraindications for vagal nerve stimulation placement EXCEPT:
   A. Upper cranial nerve deficits
   B. Presence of a single vagus nerve only
   C. Cardiac arrhythmias
   D. Lung disease
   E. Ulcers

20. The anterior loop of the internal carotid artery lies in the floor of this triangle.
   A. Lateral triangle
   B. Anterior lateral triangle
   C. Parkinson's triangle
   D. Anterior medial triangle
   E. None of the above

21. Jitter is best described as
   A. synchronous muscle fiber activation between fibers of different motor units.
   B. a difference in timing of muscle fiber activation between two fibers in a single motor unit.
   C. a difference in timing of muscle fiber activation between two fibers of different motor units.
   D. the complete failure of neuromuscular transmission at one muscle fiber in a pair.
   E. None of the above

22. Ataxia may be seen in all of the following syndromes EXCEPT:
   A. Claude's syndrome
   B. Benedikt's syndrome
   C. Nothnagel's syndrome
   D. Basilar artery syndrome
   E. Weber's syndrome

23. Which of the following is the least common complication of vagal nerve stimulation placement in the pediatric population?
    A. Hoarseness
    B. Coughing
    C. Shortness of breath
    D. Nausea
    E. Increased drooling

24. A lesion of which of the following structures would most significantly impair memory?
    A. Amygdala
    B. Fornix
    C. Dorsomedial nucleus of the thalamus
    D. Mammillary body
    E. Area 44

25. Which of the following is NOT associated with the findings on this X-ray?

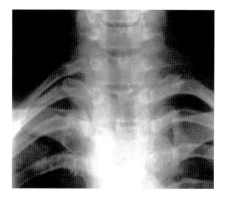

    A. Weakness of hand intrinsic flexors
    B. Horner's syndrome
    C. Raynaud's syndrome
    D. Traction meningocele
    E. Ulnar paresthesias

26. Bannayan–Riley–Ruvalcaba syndrome is associated with all the following EXCEPT:
    A. Multiple subcutaneous lipomas
    B. Macrocephaly
    C. Hemangiomas
    D. Intracranial arteriovenous malformations
    E. Capillary malformation or "port-wine stain"

27. Where is the extreme capsule located?
- **A.** Between the claustrum and the putamen
- **B.** Between the claustrum and the insular cortex
- **C.** Between the putamen and the globus pallidus externus
- **D.** Between the globus pallidus externus and the globus pallidus internus
- **E.** Above the caudate nucleus

28. Which of the following neurotransmitters promotes penile erection?
- **A.** Serotonin
- **B.** Dopamine
- **C.** Noradrenaline
- **D.** All of the above
- **E.** None of the above

29. The peak reduction in intracranial pressure (ICP) after administration of mannitol occurs in about
- **A.** 4 hours.
- **B.** 2 hours.
- **C.** 1 hour.
- **D.** 30 minutes.
- **E.** 15 minutes.

30. The borders of the paramedial triangle are cranial nerves
- **A.** I and II.
- **B.** II and III.
- **C.** III and IV.
- **D.** IV and V.
- **E.** None of the above

31. The Tensilon test
- **A.** is not sensitive but very specific for myasthenia gravis (MG).
- **B.** is not particularly useful in ocular MG.
- **C.** when negative, rules out the diagnosis of MG.
- **D.** shows no correlation with subsequent response to pyridostigmine.
- **E.** is not affected by the quantity of acetylcholine receptors.

32. In posterior interosseous syndrome, there is a fingerdrop but no wristdrop because of sparing of the
- **A.** extensor carpi radialis longus.
- **B.** extensor carpi radialis brevis.
- **C.** extensor digitorum.
- **D.** extensor carpi ulnaris.
- **E.** brachioradialis.

33. What is the Spetzler–Martin grade of this arteriovenous malformation (AVM) found in a 30-year-old asymptomatic healthy patient?

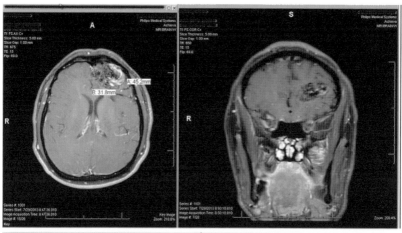

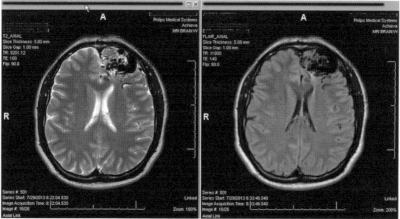

    A. 1
    B. 2
    C. 3
    D. 4
    E. 5

34. Interruption of the inferior geniculocalcarine fibers results in which of the following?
    A. Ipsilateral superior quadrantanopia
    B. Contralateral superior quadrantanopia
    C. Ipsilateral inferior quadrantanopia
    D. Contralateral inferior quadrantanopia
    E. None of the above

35. Which of the following may be seen with ocular myoclonus?
   A. Vertical oscillation of the eyes occurring with movements of the palate
   B. Hypertrophy of the inferior olivary nucleus
   C. Prior lesions of the central tegmental tract
   D. All of the above
   E. None of the above

36. All of the following characterize Acute respiratory distress syndrome (ARDS) EXCEPT:
   A. Late hypoxemia
   B. Diffuse infiltrate
   C. Leaky capillaries
   D. Association with sepsis and trauma
   E. Protein content of fluid greater than with pulmonary edema

37. In a healing wound, maximum collagen deposition occurs at
   A. 2 weeks.
   B. 4 weeks.
   C. 6 weeks.
   D. 8 weeks.
   E. 10 weeks.

38. All of the following are true regarding the condition depicted by this histopathology EXCEPT:

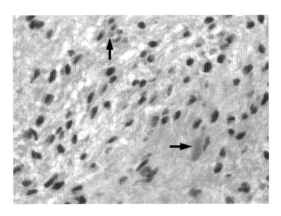

   A. It is histologically characterized by a biphasic pattern.
   B. Rosenthal fibers are a prerequisite for this diagnosis.
   C. It may mimic oligodendroglioma.
   D. It is a CNS neoplasm seen with neurofibromatosis type 1.
   E. Recurrence is usually a reformation of the cyst rather than the solid tumor.

39. Barbiturates presumably act by which of the following mechanisms?
   A. Inverse steal phenomenon
   B. Decrease CMR
   C. Decrease oxygen consumption
   D. Scavenge free radicals
   E. All of the above

40. Parkinson's (infratrochlear) triangle is defined by cranial nerves
   A. II and III.
   B. III and IV.
   C. IV and V_1.
   D. V_1 and V_2.
   E. V_2 and V_3.

41. Which of the following is true of myasthenia gravis?
   A. The majority of acetylcholine receptor antibodies are of the M subtype.
   B. Cyclosporine is used as a first-line treatment.
   C. Corticosteroids may reduce the risk of secondary generalization in the ocular form.
   D. Pathological abnormalities of the thymus are found in less than 5% of patients.
   E. Weakness confined to the ocular muscles beyond 3 years is associated with poor prognosis.

42. The border of the foramen lacerum is formed by the
   A. sphenoid bone.
   B. temporal bone.
   C. sphenoid and temporal bones.
   D. sphenoid, temporal, and occipital bones.
   E. occipital bone.

43. Absence of inflammation is typical of the following diseases EXCEPT:
   A. Neuropathy from diphtheria
   B. Creutzfeldt–Jakob disease
   C. Paraneoplastic necrotizing myelopathy
   D. Central pontine myelinolysis
   E. Tolosa–Hunt syndrome

44. Wernicke's area is BEST described as including
   A. area 39.
   B. supramarginal, area 40, and posterior one-third of the superior temporal gyri.
   C. angular and posterior one-third of the superior temporal gyri.
   D. areas 39 and 40.
   E. supramarginal and posterior one-third of the superior temporal gyri.

45. Anti-pause cell antibody may be seen with childhood infections or paraneoplastic syndrome in adults. Immune-mediated defects in pause cell function most likely result in
  A. opsoclonus.
  B. square wave jerks.
  C. downbeat nystagmus.
  D. upbeat nystagmus.
  E. None of the above

46. The origin of axons that mediate the swallowing reflex is the
  A. solitary nucleus.
  B. dorsal motor nucleus of X.
  C. nucleus ambiguus.
  D. All of the above
  E. None of the above

Match these MRI scan findings with the following comments:

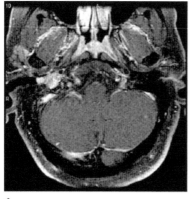
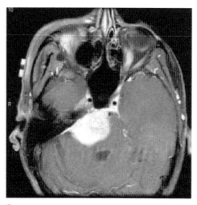

1   **2**

  A. Scan 1
  B. Scan 2
  C. Both scans 1 and 2
  D. Neither scan 1 nor scan 2

47. Hypertension

48. Early facial nerve involvement

49. Hypotension and bronchoconstriction during resection

50. Explosive diarrhea

51.   Early hearing loss and tinnitus

52.   Laboratory manifestations of disseminated intravascular coagulation (DIC) include all of the following EXCEPT:
    A.   Increased fibrinogen level
    B.   Prolonged PT
    C.   Prolonged PTT
    D.   Thrombocytopenia
    E.   Fragmented RBCs

53.   The mastoid air cells are innervated by
    A. V_1.
    B. V_2.
    C. V_3.
    D.   IX.
    E.   X.

54.   Which of the following statements is most accurate regarding the band of Gennari?
    A.   It divides the third layer of the cortex of areas 17 and 18.
    B.   It divides the third layer of the cortex of area 17.
    C.   It divides the fourth layer of the cortex of areas 17 and 18.
    D.   It divides the fourth layer of the cortex of area 17.
    E.   It divides the fourth layer of the cortex of areas 17, 18, and 19.

55.   The following are prenuclear structures for vertical gaze EXCEPT:
    A.   Nucleus of Darkshevich
    B.   Posterior commissure
    C.   Interstitial nucleus of Cajal
    D.   Rostral interstitial nucleus of the medial longitudinal fasciculus (MLF)
    E.   Nucleus prepositus hypoglossi

56.   Which of the following neurons or nerve cell processes is/are particularly involved with new, novel movements?
    A.   Mossy fibers
    B.   Betz cell
    C.   Climbing fibers
    D.   All of the above
    E.   None of the above

57. Which of the following disease states is characterized by high trophic hormone and low target hormone?
A. Cushing's disease
B. Graves's disease
C. Adrenal tumors
D. Addison's disease
E. None of the above

58. Which of the following intrinsic muscles of the thumb does NOT insert on the proximal phalanx?
A. Adductor pollicis
B. Abductor pollicis brevis
C. Flexor pollicis brevis
D. Opponens pollicis
E. Extensor pollicis brevis

59. Which of the following statements is FALSE with regard to the scan shown here?

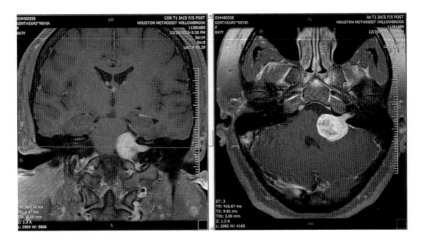

A. The first symptom in 90% of patients is unilateral hearing loss.
B. Headaches, clumsy gait, and mental confusion may occur.
C. The seventh cranial nerve is frequently involved preoperatively.
D. Essentially everyone who has been treated for an acoustic neuroma experiences difficulty with balance and/or dizziness to some degree.
E. Sporadic defects in tumor suppressor genes may give rise to these tumors.

Match these brachial plexus structures with the appropriate letter in the diagram:

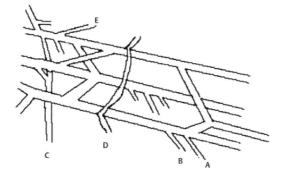

60. Medial brachial cutaneous nerve

61. Long thoracic nerve

62. Medial antebrachial cutaneous nerve

63. Suprascapular nerve

64. Median pectoral nerve

65. The medial longitudinal fasciculus (MLF) is responsible for the binocular coordination of the following eye movements EXCEPT:
A. Lateral
B. Vertical
C. Vergence
D. Oblique
E. Horizontal

66. Which of the following is a distinguishing factor between Apert's and Crouzon's syndrome?
A. Pattern of inheritance
B. Association with bilateral coronal synostosis
C. Severity of mental retardation
D. All of the above
E. None of the above

67. TRH is a secretagogue for
A. prolactin.
B. ACTH.
C. GH.
D. TSH.
E. All of the above

68. Which of the following nerves is responsible for movement of the ring finger?
  A. Radial only
  B. Radial and median
  C. Radial, median, and ulnar
  D. Radial, median, and axillary
  E. Musculocutaneous, median, and ulnar

69. Which of the following immunohistochemical profiles has been shown to be expressed in 100% of primary glioblastoma?
  A. Survivin
  B. MMP-9
  C. EGFR
  D. MDM2
  E. Fas (APO-1/CD95)

70. This triangle is defined laterally by the greater superficial petrosal nerve and medially by the petrosal sinus.
  A. Lateral triangle
  B. Paramedial triangle
  C. Glasscock's triangle
  D. Kawase's triangle
  E. Parkinson's triangle

71. Which is FALSE regarding the hormone prolactin (PRL)?
  A. Its releasing hormone is located in the arcuate nucleus.
  B. Normal levels are 5–25 ng per mL.
  C. Levels may be increased after syncope.
  D. Levels are increased after tonic clonic seizure activity.
  E. Levels are increased after nonepileptic seizures.

72. Which of the following circumventricular organs is a central receptor site for angiotensin II?
  A. Organum vasculosum of the lamina terminalis
  B. Median eminence of the tuber cinereum
  C. Subcommissural organ
  D. Subfornical organ
  E. Area postrema

73. All of the following are true of the sinuvertebral nerve EXCEPT:
  A. It is a branch from the posterior division of the spinal nerve proximal to the dorsal root ganglion.
  B. It may enter the intervertebral foramen.
  C. It supplies most of the innervation to the posterior aspect of the disk.
  D. It may have a proprioceptive and/or nociceptive function.
  E. It has been shown to consist of two roots at cervical levels.

74. All of the following are true of conduction aphasia EXCEPT:
- **A.** It is caused by a lesion of the arcuate fasciculus.
- **B.** There is fluent paraphasic speech with intact repetition.
- **C.** It may be caused by occlusion of a middle cerebral artery(MCA) posterior temporal branch.
- **D.** Patients may mimic Wernicke's disease, but are able to understand.
- **E.** Patients are aware of the problem.

75. Which statement is true about the aneurysm shown here?

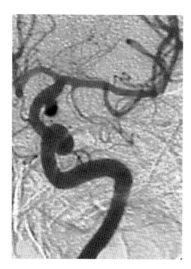

- **A.** It arises from the cavernous internal carotid artery.
- **B.** It measures ~6–8 mm.
- **C.** It usually presents pituitary dysfunction.
- **D.** All of the above statements are true.
- **E.** None of the above statements are true.

76. What does the Torg-Pavlov ratio measure?
- **A.** Vertebral blood flow
- **B.** Carotid blood flow
- **C.** Cervical stenosis
- **D.** Thoracic stenosis
- **E.** Lumbar stenosis

77. Which of the following is FALSE when comparing primary and secondary glioblastoma?
- **A.** Primary glioblastoma has an incidence that is about 10 times higher than secondary glioblastoma.
- **B.** The mean age at presentation in primary glioblastoma is much younger (45 years) than in secondary glioblastoma (62 years).
- **C.** Primary glioblastoma is more common in males when compared with secondary glioblastoma.
- **D.** The median survival at presentation is longer in secondary glioblastoma as compared with primary glioblastoma.
- **E.** Loss of heterozygosity on 10p or 10q is one of the most common genetic mutations in primary glioblastoma.

78. Cell bodies of nerve fibers in the medial brachial cutaneous nerve are found in the
- **A.** dorsal root ganglia only.
- **B.** anterior horn only.
- **C.** sympathetic chain ganglia and dorsal root ganglia.
- **D.** lateral horn and sympathetic chain ganglia.
- **E.** None of the above

79. The perforant path is the main
- **A.** inhibitory pathway of the hippocampus.
- **B.** excitatory pathway of the hippocampus.
- **C.** inhibitory pathway of the hypothalamus.
- **D.** excitatory pathway of the hypothalamus.
- **E.** None of the above

80. Which triangle has its base at the petrous apex?
- **A.** Parkinson's triangle
- **B.** Kawase's triangle
- **C.** Glasscock's triangle
- **D.** Inferior medial triangle
- **E.** Paramedial triangle

81. The most common type of headache is
- **A.** cluster.
- **B.** tension.
- **C.** migraine.
- **D.** postconcussive.
- **E.** due to temporal arteritis.

82. The trochlear nerve can be found in which cistern?
 A. Cerebellomedullary
 B. Interpeduncular
 C. Ambient
 D. Chiasmatic
 E. Pontine

83. Which scalene muscle(s) insert on the first rib?
 A. Anterior scalene
 B. Anterior and medial
 C. Medial and posterior
 D. Anterior and posterior
 E. Anterior, medial, and posterior

84. A lesion of the left geniculocalcarine tract and the corpus callosum is most likely to cause
 A. pure word blindness.
 B. pure word deafness.
 C. mutism.
 D. anomic aphasia.
 E. global aphasia.

85. All of the following are true regarding hemispherectomy EXCEPT:
 A. Improvement in IQ is often seen postoperatively.
 B. Behavior is improved after surgery.
 C. It is not necessary to preserve the septum pellucidum.
 D. The foramen of Monro is often plugged with a piece of temporalis muscle.
 E. Patients are usually uncommunicative for about a week after surgery.

86. The principle behind multiple subpial transection for epilepsy is that
 A. horizontal fibers have a limited functional role.
 B. vertical fibers have a limited functional role.
 C. the pia has a limited functional role.
 D. All of the above
 E. None of the above

87. The presenting symptom of a hypothalamic hamartoma is most commonly
 A. headache.
 B. vomiting.
 C. visual field disturbance.
 D. sexual precocity.
 E. seizures.

88.   All of the following are true of the tumor in this pathology slide EXCEPT:

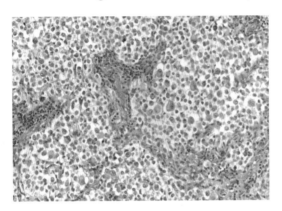

    A.   It is found in superficial brain regions.
    B.   It shows intracellular accumulation of lipids.
    C.   It corresponds to WHO grade II.
    D.   It carries a dismal prognosis.
    E.   It presents in patients with a long history of seizures.

89.   Schaffer collaterals carry
    A.   excitatory input from CA1.
    B.   excitatory input from CA3.
    C.   inhibitory input from CA1.
    D.   inhibitory input from CA3.
    E.   None of the above

90.   Which of the following muscles would you expect to find weak given the finding on this scan?

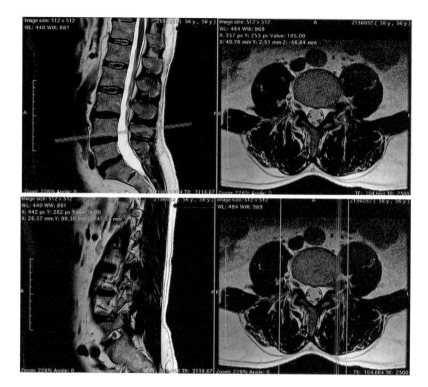

A.   Gastrocnemius
B.   Tibialis anterior
C.   Extensor hallucis longus
D.   Iliopsoas
E.   None of the above

91.   Which is the optimal approach for resection of the lesion in the scan shown previously for Question 90?
A.   Midline laminectomy approach
B.   Paramedian partial facetectomy approach
C.   Transforaminal lumbar interbody fusion
D.   Posterior lumbar interbody fusion
E.   A and C

92.   All of the following structures are supplied by the anterior spinal artery EXCEPT:
A.   Pyramids
B.   Medial lemniscus
C.   Fibers of cranial nerve XII
D.   Gracile and cuneate nuclei
E.   Anterior two-thirds of the spinal cord

93. During a clinic appointment, the patient is asked to sit with the arms dependent, hold her breath, and tilt her head back and turn it to the side. Meanwhile the doctor is checking for presence or absence of a radial pulse. What is being described?
A. Allen's test
B. Ayer's test
C. Adson's test
D. Addis test
E. Dix–Hallpike maneuver

94. The corticobulbar tract is located in which area of the internal capsule?
A. Anterior limb
B. Posterior limb
C. Retrolenticular limb
D. Sublenticular limb
E. Genu

95. The medial forebrain bundle interconnects the following areas EXCEPT:
A. Septal nuclei
B. Raphe nuclei
C. Locus ceruleus
D. Medulla
E. Hypothalamus

96. Cerebellar tonsillar displacement is seen in
A. Chiari I.
B. Chiari II.
C. Crouzon's syndrome.
D. All of the above
E. None of the above

97. The most severe forms of hypothalamic cachexia are seen in lesions of the
A. lateral hypothalamus.
B. anterior hypothalamus.
C. posterior hypothalamus.
D. ventromedial hypothalamus.
E. suprachiasmatic hypothalamus.

98. The region of the cortex most closely associated with the conscious perception of smell is the
A. temporal cortex.
B. cingulate cortex.
C. prefrontal cortex.
D. posterior parietal cortex.
E. anterior parietal cortex.

99. Which amino acids are precursors for catecholamines?
- **A.** Phenylalanine and tyrosine
- **B.** Phenylalanine and tryptophan
- **C.** Tyrosine and tryptophan
- **D.** Arginine and tyrosine
- **E.** Phenylalanine and arginine

100. Which of the following pathological diagnoses is most likely associated with this hemorrhagic lesion?

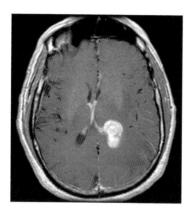

- **A.** Melanoma
- **B.** Choriocarcinoma
- **C.** Breast carcinoma
- **D.** Renal cell carcinoma
- **E.** Choroid plexus papilloma

101. In contrast to primary glioblastomas, the most common genetic mutation seen in secondary glioblastomas is
- **A.** loss of heterozygosity 10q.
- **B.** TP53 mutation.
- **C.** EGFR amplification.
- **D.** p16^{INK4a} deletion.
- **E.** PTEN mutations (25%).

102. The straight sinus is formed from the union of the
- **A.** internal cerebral vein and basal vein.
- **B.** inferior sagittal sinus and vein of Galen.
- **C.** basal vein and great cerebral vein.
- **D.** inferior sagittal vein and basal vein.
- **E.** precentral cerebellar vein and internal cerebral vein.

103. A lesion of the vestibular labyrinth that causes images in the visual fields to move back and forth is best described as
   A. ocular flutter.
   B. ocular dysmetria.
   C. ocular bobbing.
   D. oscillopsia.
   E. opsoclonus.

104. Atropine mainly affects which type of synapses?
   A. Parasympathetic preganglionic
   B. Parasympathetic postganglionic
   C. Sympathetic postganglionic
   D. All of the above
   E. None of the above

105. Wernicke's encephalopathy is due to deficiency of
   A. vitamin B_1.
   B. vitamin B_2.
   C. vitamin B_6.
   D. vitamin B_{12}.
   E. None of the above

106. The solitary pathways are concerned with
   A. taste.
   B. thoracic viscera.
   C. sudden changes in blood pressure.
   D. All of the above
   E. None of the above

107. The greatest difference between diffuse astrocytomas (WHO grade II) and anaplastic astrocytomas (WHO grade III) is
   A. MIB-1 fraction.
   B. the presence of mitotic activity.
   C. the presence of necrosis.
   D. angiogenesis.
   E. the presence of gemistocytes.

108. The most common intraconal orbital mass is the
   A. neurilemmoma.
   B. fibrous histiocytoma.
   C. hemangiopericytoma.
   D. cavernous hemangioma.
   E. None of the above

109. HIV-infected individuals have an increased risk of cerebrovascular events, such as stroke, when the following risk factors are present EXCEPT:
   A.   Intravenous drug abuse
   B.   Low CD4 cell count
   C.   Exposure to abacavir
   D.   Exposure to highly active antiretroviral therapy (HAART)
   E.   CD4 cell count ≤ 200 cells/μL before the start of HAART

110. The location of the apex in most arteriovenous malformations is
   A.   cortical.
   B.   insular.
   C.   parietal.
   D.   occipital.
   E.   periventricular.

111. In catecholamine biosynthesis, the rate-limiting step during conditions of neuronal activation is
   A.   dopamine β-hydroxylase.
   B.   tyrosine hydroxylase.
   C.   aromatic amino acid decarboxylase.
   D.   monoamine oxidase.
   E.   phenylethanolamine N-methyltransferase.

112. The venous angle is seen angiographically by the junction of which two veins?
   A.   Septal and caudate
   B.   Septal and terminal
   C.   Terminal and caudate
   D.   Internal cerebral and terminal
   E.   Basal and internal cerebral

113. Ocular bobbing may be seen in which of the following?
   A.   Hydrocephalus
   B.   Pontine infarct
   C.   Hepatic encephalopathy
   D.   Trauma
   E.   All of the above

114. The most likely diagnosis for this lesion seen on CT is

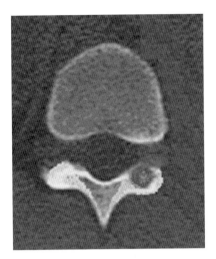

   A. aneurysmal bone cyst.
   B. epidermoid granuloma.
   C. osteosarcoma.
   D. hemangioma.
   E. osteoid osteoma.

115. The striae medullares (rhombencephali) arise from
   A. the septal nuclei.
   B. the habenular trigone.
   C. the arcuate nuclei.
   D. the amygdala.
   E. None of the above

116. The delivery of nutrients and removal of wastes from the vertebral disk is dependent on
   A. arterioles and venules.
   B. capillaries penetrating the disk.
   C. diffusion.
   D. All of the above
   E. None of the above

117. Which of the following statements is true of the olivocochlear bundle?
   A. It is part of the ascending auditory pathway to the dorsal cochlear nucleus.
   B. It can be seen readily in brainstem sections of the upper pons.
   C. It communicates directly with the medial lemniscus.
   D. Stimulation of it inhibits acoustic fiber responses to auditory stimuli.
   E. It arises from the inferior olivary nucleus and projects to the cochlea.

118. Which of the following orbital tumors is at highest risk of tumor seeding and recurrence during removal?
- **A.** Cavernous hemangioma
- **B.** Pleomorphic adenoma of the lacrimal gland
- **C.** Neurilemmoma
- **D.** Hemangiopericytoma
- **E.** Fibrous histiocytoma

119. The pterygoid plates are made up of which bones?
- **A.** Sphenoid and temporal
- **B.** Sphenoid and vomer
- **C.** Palatine and sphenoid
- **D.** Palatine
- **E.** None of the above

120. Brodmann area 44 is a part of
- **A.** Wernicke's area.
- **B.** Visual cortex.
- **C.** Broca's area.
- **D.** Prefrontal area.
- **E.** Frontal eye field.

121. Which one of the following is NOT a characteristic of hydromyelia?
- **A.** The fluid collection may communicate with the fourth ventricle.
- **B.** The fluid collection may be noncommunicating with the fourth ventricle.
- **C.** The fluid collection is typically not lined by ependymal cells.
- **D.** It may be associated with hydrocephalus.
- **E.** It may be associated with Chiari malformation.

122. Which of the following arteries supplies the deep cerebellar nuclei?
- **A.** Posterior inferior cerebellar artery
- **B.** Superior cerebellar artery
- **C.** Thalamogeniculate branches
- **D.** Posterior choroidal artery
- **E.** None of the above

123. In the comatose patient, extensor movements of the arms and weak flexor movements of the legs are most likely to occur with a lesion
- **A.** above the red nucleus.
- **B.** at the red nucleus.
- **C.** between the red nucleus and above the vestibular nuclei.
- **D.** at the vestibular nuclei.
- **E.** below the vestibular nuclei.

124. "Crocodile tears" or lacrimation from gustatory stimulation is classically described as the result of aberrant regeneration of fibers from
  A.   cranial nerve III reaching the ciliary ganglion.
  B.   cranial nerve V reaching the ciliary ganglion.
  C.   cranial nerve VII reaching the ciliary ganglion.
  D.   cranial nerve III reaching the sphenopalatine ganglion.
  E.   cranial nerve VII reaching the sphenopalatine ganglion.

125. Syringomyelia affecting the lower cervical area may result in attenuation or abolition of which of the following somatosensory evoked potentials?
  A.   N13
  B.   N20
  C.   P40
  D.   N22
  E.   None of the above

126. If an instrumentation system is too stiff, disuse osteoporosis can occur around the instrumentation. This statement is related to
  A.   Sherrington's law.
  B.   Flourens' law.
  C.   Wolff's law.
  D.   Delpech's principle.
  E.   Jackson's law.

127. In comparison to chordomas, chondrosarcomas
  A.   arise more laterally.
  B.   result in more neurological deficits at presentation.
  C.   are nearly always S-100 positive.
  D.   display all of the above features.
  E.   display none of the above features.

128. Which of the following conditions would benefit most from thalamotomy?
  A.   Medically refractory essential tremor
  B.   Rigidity associated with Parkinson's disease
  C.   Intention tremor from cerebellar stroke
  D.   Bradykinesia associated with progressive supranuclear palsy (PSP)
  E.   Dyskinesia associated with striatonigral degeneration

129. Which of the following is the best measure of the "equator" of the spinal cord when performing a cordotomy for pain management?
  A.   Just ventral to the dentate ligament
  B.   Just dorsal to the dentate ligament
  C.   At the attachment of the dentate ligament
  D.   The midway point between the exit of the dorsal and ventral rootlets
  E.   Approximately 5 mm from the anterior spinal artery

130. When is the earliest time after radiation therapy that one would expect to observe the changes appearing on this T2-weighted MRI taken in a patient who underwent a tumor resection?

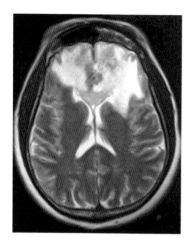

    A. 1 month
    B. 3 months
    C. 14 months
    D. 48 months
    E. 72 months

131. Levels of L-dopa are virtually unmeasurable in the central nervous system under basal conditions because
    A. the activity of tyrosine hydroxylase is low.
    B. L-dopa is localized in vesicles.
    C. the activity of aromatic amino acid decarboxylase is high.
    D. dopamine β hydroxylase is localized in the vesicles.
    E. the activity of tyrosine hydroxylase is high.

132. The facial nucleus and the spinal trigeminal nucleus and tract are supplied by which artery?
    A. Posterior inferior cerebellar artery (PICA)
    B. Anterior inferior cerebellar artery (AICA)
    C. Superior cerebellar artery (SCA)
    D. Basilar
    E. Anterior choroidal

133. Which of the following statements regarding the length constant of a nerve fiber is true?
    A. The length constant is directly proportional to the membrane resistance.
    B. It is the distance along a fiber where a change in the membrane potential by a given current decays to half its original value.
    C. The length constant is directly proportional to the axial resistance.
    D. The length constant is greater in unmyelinated than myelinated fibers.
    E. None of the above

134. Dysfunction of which cell is the main problem in Raynaud's phenomenon?
    A. Red blood cell
    B. Sympathetic neuron
    C. Platelet
    D. Mast cell
    E. Fibroblast

135. Epidural hematomas in children are the result of
    A. arterial injury.
    B. bone oozing.
    C. bleeding from the periosteal surface.
    D. All of the above
    E. None of the above

136. Spondylolysis most often occurs at
    A. L1.
    B. L2.
    C. L3.
    D. L4.
    E. L5.

137.   The finding seen in the photograph is caused by damage to

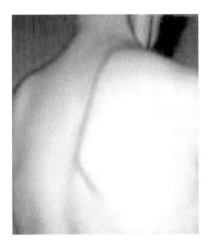

    A.   a nerve arising from the upper trunk of the brachial plexus.
    B.   a nerve arising from the roots of the brachial plexus.
    C.   the dorsal scapular nerve.
    D.   the thoracodorsal nerve.
    E.   None of the above

138.   The typical target for thalamotomy for reduction of tremor is
    A.   Vim.
    B.   Vop.
    C.   Voa.
    D.   VC.
    E.   None of the above

139.   Which of the following structures are derived from the telencephalon?
    A.   Caudate
    B.   Putamen
    C.   Amygdala
    D.   All of the above
    E.   None of the above

140.   The precuneus (Brodmann areas 7 and 31) is located
    A.   on the medial surface of the frontal lobe.
    B.   in the secondary visual cortex.
    C.   within the occipital lobe.
    D.   on the medial surface of the parietal lobe.
    E.   on the medial surface of the occipital lobe.

141. Given the imaging provided, the indications for surgery include all of the following EXCEPT:

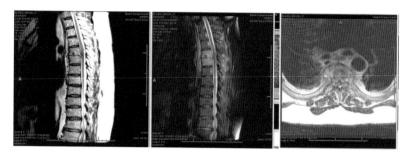

    A. Failure of medical treatment
    B. Open biopsy
    C. Significant bony or paraspinal abscess with sepsis
    D. Significant bony destruction on CT scan due to limited penetration of medical treatment
    E. Sensory deficit along the rib cage

142. Neural crest derivatives include all of the following EXCEPT:
    A. Schwann cells
    B. Bipolar cells
    C. Leptomeninges
    D. Chromaffin cells of the suprarenal medulla
    E. Parafollicular cells

143. Which of the following is located in the bony modiolus of the cochlea?
    A. Scala vestibuli
    B. Cochlear duct
    C. Organ of corti
    D. Spiral ganglion
    E. Basilar membrane

144. Damage to this area leaves the patient transiently mute, with complete recovery in a few weeks.
    A. Broca's area
    B. Wernicke's area
    C. Arcuate fasciculus
    D. Uncinate fasciculus
    E. Supplementary motor area

145. The foramen spinosum is located in
    A. the sphenoid bone anterior to the greater and lesser superficial petrosal nerves.
    B. the sphenoid bone between to the greater and lesser superficial petrosal nerves.
    C. the temporal bone posterior to the greater and lesser superficial petrosal nerves.
    D. the temporal bone between the greater and lesser superficial petrosal nerves.
    E. None of the above

146. Spondyloptosis corresponds to Meyerding grade
    A. I.
    B. II.
    C. III.
    D. IV.
    E. V.

147. Golgi tendon organs are
    A. sensitive to stretch.
    B. in series with extrafusal fibers.
    C. encapsulated.
    D. All of the above
    E. None of the above

148. During a thalamotomy procedure, which of the following indicates that the electrode is in the correct location?
    A. Low frequency (2 Hz) stimulation causes driving of the tremor.
    B. The patient reports contralateral paresthesias.
    C. High-frequency (50 Hz) stimulation results in tremor suppression.
    D. All of the above
    E. None of the above

149. Olfactory glomeruli are made up of
    A. granule and tufted cells.
    B. granule and mitral cells.
    C. tufted and mitral cells.
    D. granule cells only.
    E. None of the above

150. The sylvian triangle is defined by points along which artery/arteries?
    A. MCA only
    B. MCA and ACA
    C. ACA, MCA, and PCA
    D. MCA and PCA
    E. ACA only

151.   Select the FALSE statement regarding monoamine oxidase (MAO).
   A. MAO_A has a high affinity for norepinephrine and serotonin.
   B. MAO_A is selectively inhibited by clorgyline.
   C. MAO_B has a high affinity for o-phenylethylamines.
   D. MAO_A and MAO_B are associated with the inner mitochondrial membrane.
   E. MAO_B is selectively inhibited by deprenyl.

152.   The superior part of the fourth ventricle is derived from which of the following vesicles?
   A.   Metencephalon
   B.   Myelencephalon
   C.   Mesencephalon
   D.   Prosencephalon
   E.   None of the above

153.   This structure is a projection of the spiral limbus that overlies the hair cells of the organ of Corti.
   A.   Tectorial membrane
   B.   Basilar membrane
   C.   Vestibular membrane
   D.   Reissner's membrane
   E.   None of the above

154.   Which fibers are associated with the gag reflex?
   A.   Spinal trigeminal nucleus projections to the nucleus ambiguus
   B.   Solitary projections to the nucleus ambiguus
   C.   Solitary projections to the salivatory nucleus
   D.   Salivatory nucleus projections to the dorsal motor nucleus of the vagus
   E.   None of the above

155. A 64-year-old man presents to the clinic with severe back pain going down the left lateral leg (see X-ray). He states that the pain is worst when he reaches and bends to the right. He is most comfortable when he is lying still. He has attempted and failed conservative therapy of medication and physical therapy. If surgery is offered, what would be the best choice from the following options?

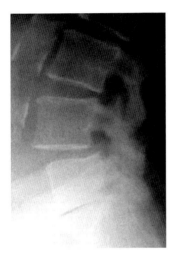

A. Lumbar laminectomy of L4–S1
B. Lumbar hemilaminectomy at L4 on left side
C. Pedicle screw fusion of L4–L5
D. Pedicle screw fusion of L3–S1
E. Pedicle screw fusion of L3–L4

156. Which of the following receptors is activated by baclofen and is insensitive to bicuculline?
A. GABA-A
B. GABA-B
C. GABA-C
D. All of the above
E. None of the above

157. All of the following structures pass through the annulus of Zinn (tendinous ring) EXCEPT:
A. Cranial nerve III, superior division
B. Nasociliary nerve
C. Cranial nerve IV
D. Cranial nerve III, inferior division
E. Cranial nerve VI

Match the organisms associated with the lesion shown here, given the patient presentation:

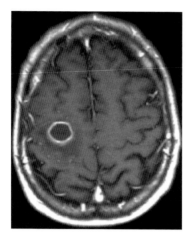

    A. *Proteus*
    B. *Streptococcus*
    C. *Staphylococcus*
    D. *Pseudomonas*

158. Sixteen year-old boy who sustained a parietal skull fracture after a motorcycle accident

159. Sixty-year-old woman with chronic ear infection

160. Three-month-old baby with irritability and decreased oral intake

161. Tranylcypromine is
    A. an inhibitor of MAO_A.
    B. an inhibitor of MAO_B.
    C. an inhibitor of COMT.
    D. a reuptake inhibitor of serotonin.
    E. an inhibitor of acetylcholinesterase.

162. Which is the embryological structure that becomes the ventral white commissure in the adult?
    A. Basal plate
    B. Floor plate
    C. Alar plate
    D. Basal plate
    E. Sulcus limitans

163. Which of the following is FALSE regarding the syndrome that has a prominent feature illustrated in this CT scan?

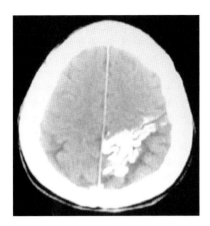

    A.   There is involvement of the upper eyelid.
    B.   Radiotherapy is not effective.
    C.   Hemiparesis is contralateral to the facial lesion.
    D.   The triad classically consists of nevus flammeus, venous malformation, and glaucoma.
    E.   Abnormalities of chromosome 9 are seen.

164. CSF is produced by
    A.   choroid plexus.
    B.   ependymal surface.
    C.   brain parenchyma.
    D.   bulk flow from the brain.
    E.   All of the above

165. In patients with known systemic cancer, what percentage of single brain lesions are cerebral abscesses or primary brain tumors?
    A.   Less than 0.1%
    B.   1%
    C.   15%
    D.   30%
    E.   50%

166. Vigabatrin has anticonvulsant properties related to its interference of
    A.   GABA breakdown.
    B.   GABA synthesis.
    C.   GABA reuptake.
    D.   All of the above
    E.   None of the above

167. The indusium griseum is a remnant of
   A.   the habenula.
   B.   the hippocampus.
   C.   the hypothalamus.
   D.   the gyrus of Heschl.
   E.   None of the above

168. A patient who had a thalamotomy for Parkinsonian tremor earlier in the month has noticed weakness of the arm. The most likely explanation for this is that the lesion placed during the thalamotomy was too
   A.   medial.
   B.   lateral.
   C.   anterior.
   D.   posterior.
   E.   mild.

169. Which immunosuppressive agent works at the level of the T cells by inhibiting expression of interleukin (IL)-2?
   A.   Azathioprine
   B.   Cyclosporine
   C.   Methotrexate
   D.   All of the above
   E.   None of the above

170. Posterior thalamo-perforating arteries are the perforators that arise from which artery?
   A.   Pcom
   B.   Pcom and P1
   C.   P1 and P2
   D.   P2
   E.   P1

171. Which nucleus of the hypothalamus gives rise to dopamine innervation of the median eminence?
   A.   Supraoptic
   B.   Dorsomedial
   C.   Lateral
   D.   Arcuate
   E.   Ventromedial

172. The alar plate gives rise to all of the following EXCEPT:
   A.   Gracile and cuneate nuclei
   B.   Inferior olivary nuclei
   C.   Solitary nucleus
   D.   Spinal trigeminal nucleus
   E.   Nucleus ambiguus

173. Normal thoracic kyphosis is generally accepted to vary from
   A. 10–35°.
   B. 20–45°.
   C. 30–55°.
   D. 40–65°.
   E. 50–70°.

174. In preparation for placement of a ventriculostomy catheter, a resident measures a point 2.5 cm from the midline and 1 cm anterior to the coronal suture. The point that is being measured is
   A. Keen's point.
   B. Kocher's point.
   C. McEwen's point.
   D. Barker's point.
   E. Sylvian point.

175. A 60-year-old man with this MRI finding is most likely to present with the following signs on examination:

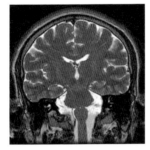 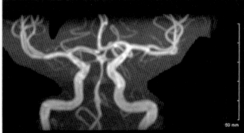

   A. Bilateral limb ataxia
   B. Ipsilateral Horner's syndrome
   C. Contralateral abducens palsy
   D. Ipsilateral tongue paralysis
   E. None of the above

176. All of the following epilepsy drugs have hepatic enzyme-inducing properties EXCEPT:
   A. Carbamazepine
   B. Phenytoin
   C. Clonazepam
   D. Primidone
   E. Phenobarbitone

177. The interposed nuclei project to
    A.   the contralateral red nucleus.
    B.   the ipsilateral red nucleus.
    C.   the contralateral thalamus.
    D.   the ipsilateral thalamus.
    E.   None of the above

178. All of the following symptoms may improve after pallidotomy EXCEPT:
    A.   Drug-induced dyskinesias
    B.   Painful dystonias
    C.   On/off fluctuations
    D.   Bradykinesia
    E.   Postural instability

179. With regard to neurological manifestations of HIV disease, which of the following is true?
    A.   Neurological involvement in HIV infection is more frequent in adults than in children.
    B.   Neurological complications occur in less than 20% of patients with HIV infection.
    C.   Neurological complications are the presenting feature of AIDS in 20% of cases.
    D.   At autopsy, the prevalence of neuropathological abnormalities is ~20%.
    E.   An ongoing increase in HIV-associated CNS disease has been observed in very recent years

180. AICA originates from the
    A.   vertebral artery.
    B.   distal one-third of the vertebral artery.
    C.   proximal two-thirds of the basilar artery.
    D.   posterior cerebral artery.
    E.   distal two-thirds of the basilar artery.

181. Which is FALSE regarding serotonin?
    A.   It is metabolized to melatonin in the pineal gland.
    B.   The majority of body stores of serotonin are found in the central nervous system.
    C.   Two critical enzymes take part in its synthesis.
    D.   Tryptophan is the precursor amino acid.
    E.   It has an indole structure.

182. The basal plate gives rise to all of the following EXCEPT:
    A.   Oculomotor nucleus
    B.   Trochlear nucleus
    C.   Substantia nigra
    D.   Red nucleus
    E.   Superior colliculus

183. Which of the following are more expressed in painful degenerative disk disease as compared with disk herniation?
    A. Tumor necrosis factor-α and interleukin (IL)-8
    B. IL-1β and IL-6
    C. IL-6 and IL-12
    D. IL-3 and IL-4
    E. None of the above

184. During the abdominal portion of the operation for a ventroperitoneal (VP) shunt, if the surgeon is below the arcuate line, which structures would lie behind the rectus abdominis?
    A. External oblique aponeurosis
    B. Internal oblique aponeurosis
    C. Transversus abdominis aponeurosis
    D. Transversalis fascia
    E. None of the above

185. Which of the following posterior fossa tumors has the tendency to arise from the floor of the fourth ventricle?
    A. Medulloblastoma
    B. Ependymoma
    C. Astrocytoma
    D. Hemangioblastoma
    E. None of the above

186. Which of the following is true of Lissauer's tract?
    A. Its fibers are derived from the lateral division of the dorsal roots.
    B. It contains Aδ fibers.
    C. It contains C fibers.
    D. All of the above
    E. None of the above

187. The limen insula can be found
    A. in the occipital lobe.
    B. at the junction of the insula and the frontal lobe.
    C. within the third ventricle.
    D. in cross sections through the pons.
    E. in none of the above.

188. During pallidotomy when the surgeon believes the electrode is near the target, a high-frequency stimulation is performed to insure that the electrode is not too close to the
    A. thalamus.
    B. internal capsule.
    C. optic tract.
    D. amygdala.
    E. putamen.

189. The apex of the thoracic curvature typically lies at
   A. T3.
   B. T5.
   C. T7.
   D. T9.
   E. T11.

190. An important landmark for identifying the junction of the tegmentum and the cerebral peduncle is the
   A. anterior pontomesencephalic vein.
   B. lateral mesencephalic vein.
   C. precentral cerebellar vein.
   D. vein of Galen.
   E. superior vermian vein.

191. This amino acid is not only a precursor to GABA but is also a neurotransmitter.
   A. Glycine
   B. Glutamate
   C. Arginine
   D. Tyrosine
   E. Tryptophan

192. Which of the following is FALSE regarding stiff person syndrome?
   A. It is transmitted in an autosomal recessive pattern.
   B. The stiffness primarily affects the truncal muscles.
   C. Chronic pain and impaired mobility are common symptoms.
   D. Lumbar hyperlordosis is often seen.
   E. Patients have high glutamic acid decarboxylase antibody titers.

193. All of the following inflammatory factors are expressed at high levels in degenerative disk disease EXCEPT:
   A. Interleukin (IL)-1β
   B. IL-3
   C. IL-6
   D. IL-8
   E. Tumor necrosis factor-α

194. In phenylketonuria, the deficiency of phenylalanine hydroxylase results in decreased levels of
   A. dopamine.
   B. norepinephrine.
   C. serotonin.
   D. None of the above
   E. All of the above

195. Classic phenylketonuria is characterized by all EXCEPT:
  A. Low levels of prolactin
  B. Increased gray matter volume in the ventral part of the striatum
  C. A diet low in phenylalanine as a major part of disease management
  D. Neurological symptoms such as intellectual disability, tremors, seizures, and jerky movements
  E. Occurs in 1 in 10,000 to 15,000 newborns

196. Which of the following findings is LEAST likely to be associated with this MRI scan?

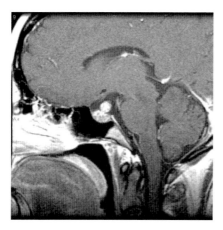

  A. Elevated serum angiotensin-converting enzyme
  B. Eosinophilic granuloma
  C. Meningitis
  D. Elevated adrenocorticotrophic hormone
  E. Sarcoidosis

197. A central facial palsy would involve
  A. only the ipsilateral upper face.
  B. only the ipsilateral lower face.
  C. only the contralateral upper face.
  D. only the contralateral lower face.
  E. None of the above

198. Palatal nystagmus is most likely due to a lesion of
  A. the dorsal spinocerebellar tract.
  B. the corticospinal tract.
  C. the middle cerebellar peduncle.
  D. the central tegmental tract.
  E. None of the above

199. The single best predictor for patients with esthesioneuroblastoma is
    A.   completeness of primary tumor excision and extent of involvement at presentation.
    B.   TP53 overexpression.
    C.   the presence of Homer–Wright rosettes on pathology.
    D.   neuron-specific enolase expression.
    E.   destruction of the cribriform plate.

200. During a lateral suboccipital approach for tumor resection, cerebellar retraction may be excessive if the BSAEP indicates
    A.   increased latency in wave 3.
    B.   decreased latency in wave 4.
    C.   decreased latency in wave 5.
    D.   increased latency in wave 4.
    E.   increased latency in wave 5.

201. The best-characterized glutamate-containing neurons are found in the
    A.   Purkinje cells of the cerebellum.
    B.   pyramidal cells of the cerebral cortex.
    C.   pyramidal cells of the hippocampus.
    D.   septal region.
    E.   lateral entorhinal cortex.

202. All of the following statements are true of nuclear chain fibers EXCEPT:
    A.   They receive group Ia primary afferent fibers.
    B.   They receive group II secondary afferent fibers.
    C.   They are associated with flower spray endings.
    D.   They are associated with static gamma efferent fibers.
    E.   They respond to muscle tension.

203. Patients who continue to display mental status changes after correction of diabetic ketoacidosis should be investigated for
    A.   cysticercosis.
    B.   histoplasmosis.
    C.   Lyme disease.
    D.   mucormycosis.
    E.   hydatid disease.

204. Which of the following is FALSE with regard to shunt nephritis?
    A.   It is a well-described complication of VP shunts.
    B.   It is due to deposition of immune complexes in the glomeruli of kidneys.
    C.   The diagnosis is suspected with hematuria, elevated erythrocyte sedimentation rate (ESR), and decreased complement levels.
    D.   Proper treatment entails removing the entire shunt.
    E.   There is an elevated peripheral WBC count.

205. Regarding DNET, which of the following is FALSE?
  A. Male predominance has been noted.
  B. It is a surgically curable cause of partial seizures.
  C. There is an abundance of mitoses with no necrosis.
  D. It is a mixed glial and neuronal neoplasm.
  E. It shows on CT scans as a hypodense pseudocystic lesion.

206. Which of the following is the most appropriate next step in management of a hypertensive patient who sustained recurrent falling episodes and complains of headache with the MRI findings shown here?

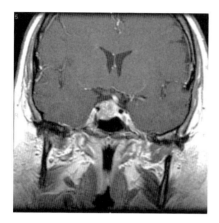

  A. Transsphenoidal resection
  B. Bromocriptine
  C. Angiography
  D. Ophthalmologic evaluation
  E. Transcranial resection

207. The saccule sends fibers to the _____vestibular ganglion which project to the _____vestibular nucleus.
  A. Superior, superior
  B. Superior, inferior
  C. Inferior, superior
  D. Inferior, inferior
  E. None of the above

208. Which of the following tracts traverse the restiform body?
  A. Olivocerebellar
  B. Reticulocerebellar
  C. Dorsal spinocerebellar
  D. All of the above
  E. None of the above

209. A favorable prognosis in neuroblastomas is related to
    A. n-Myc amplification.
    B. 1p deletion.
    C. TrkA expression.
    D. older age.
    E. None of the above

210. For microvascular decompression in a patient with trigeminal neuralgia, the first bur hole is best placed at the
    A. mastoid tip.
    B. key hole.
    C. asterion.
    D. bregma.
    E. lambda.

211. The definitive marker for cholinergic neurons is
    A. acetyl CoA.
    B. acetylcholinesterase.
    C. choline acetyltransferase.
    D. choline.
    E. sensitivity to hemicholinium-3.

212. Tanycytes are most likely to be found in
    A. the wall of the third ventricle.
    B. a high-grade glioma.
    C. a low-grade glioma.
    D. the cauda equina.
    E. None of the above

Match the statement with the appropriate structure on the diagram:

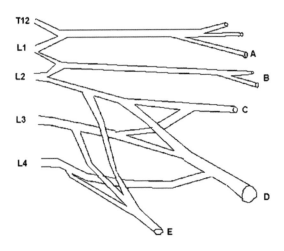

213.   Genitofemoral nerve

214.   Innervates the sartorius muscle

215.   Enables leg abduction

216.   Meralgia paresthetica

217.   The vagus nerve leaves the medulla
   A.   between the pyramid and the olive.
   B.   between the olive and the inferior cerebellar peduncle.
   C.   from the same sulcus as CN XII.
   D.   from the dorsomedial sulcus.
   E.   from none of the above.

218.   Bilateral damage to the medial basal occipitotemporal cortex results in
   A.   astereognosis.
   B.   prosoprognosia.
   C.   alexia without agraphia.
   D.   auditory agnosia.
   E.   autotopagnosia.

219.   Neuroblastomas may present with
   A.   spinal cord compression.
   B.   Ondine's curse.
   C.   opsoclonus syndrome.
   D.   diarrhea.
   E.   All of the above

220.   One of the most significant prognostic indicators for successful prolactinoma surgery is
   A.   the results of the Goldman perimetry field.
   B.   being male.
   C.   the preoperative prolactin level.
   D.   the age of the patient.
   E.   being female.

221.   Nitric oxide synthase is responsible for
   A.   conversion of R-arginine into nitrous oxide (NO).
   B.   conversion of citrulline into NO.
   C.   production of NO and L-arginine.
   D.   production of NO and citrulline.
   E.   None of the above

222. Which Rexed lamina is homologous to the spinal trigeminal tract?
- **A.** I
- **B.** II
- **C.** III and IV
- **D.** VII
- **E.** IX

223. The most common presentation of vein of Galen malformation in the neonate is
- **A.** an intracranial bruit with heart failure.
- **B.** subarachnoid hemorrhage.
- **C.** hydrocephalus.
- **D.** developmental delay.
- **E.** ocular symptoms.

224. Which of the following associations based on this MRI scan is FALSE?

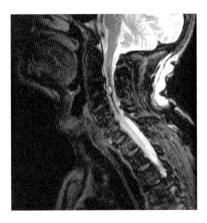

- **A.** Subarachnoid hemorrhage
- **B.** Progressive ascending paraplegic syndrome
- **C.** The definitive therapy is microsurgical elimination.
- **D.** Tendency to bleed in elderly patients
- **E.** It may represent a vascular anomaly.

225. The arcuate eminence is the bony landmark of
- **A.** the superior petrosal sinus.
- **B.** the superior semicircular canal.
- **C.** the middle meningeal artery.
- **D.** the vein of Labbé.
- **E.** None of the above

226. Which of the following is true of the medial posterior choroidal artery?
   A.   It is a branch of the posterior cerebral artery.
   B.   It supplies the choroid plexus of the third ventricle.
   C.   It supplies the choroid plexus of the lateral ventricles.
   D.   All of the above
   E.   None of the above

227. The calamus scriptorius can be found
   A.   in the third ventricle.
   B.   in the fourth ventricle.
   C.   in the lateral ventricle.
   D.   at the cauda equina.
   E.   in none of the above.

228. Brain waves that are characteristic of deep sleep and have a frequency of 1 to 3 per second are
   A.   α waves.
   B.   β waves.
   C.   theta waves.
   D.   delta waves.
   E.   None of the above

229. Which cranial nerves innervate muscles that attach to the styloid process?
   A.   VII, IX, X
   B.   IX, X
   C.   IX, X, XII
   D.   VII, X
   E.   VII, IX, XII

230. The sagittal vertical axis offset is a measure of sagittal balance performed by using the following:
   A.   C7 plumb line
   B.   Cobb angle
   C.   Pelvic tilt
   D.   Sacral slope
   E.   None of the above

231. Allodynia is a condition in which
   A.   a painful response is produced by an innocuous mechanical stimulus.
   B.   a painful response is felt in an amputated limb.
   C.   a painful response is felt on the opposite side of the body.
   D.   there is sensitization of spinocerebellar neurons.
   E.   all of the above may occur.

232.   The nucleus dorsalis of Clarke corresponds to which Rexed lamina?
   A.   I
   B.   II
   C.   III and IV
   D.   VII
   E.   IX

233.   All of the following are true of encephaloceles EXCEPT:
   A.   Occipital encephaloceles are the most common type.
   B.   Frontoethmoidal (sincipital) are the most common type in southeast Asia and among Australian aborigines.
   C.   Parietal encephaloceles are associated with Chiari II malformation in up to one-third of cases.
   D.   Basal encephaloceles are associated with defects along the sphenoid bone.
   E.   Children with basal encephaloceles have a low risk of developing meningitis.

234.   On a horizontal section of the brain, the anterior limb of the internal capsule can be found between
   A.   the thalamus and the globus pallidus.
   B.   the caudate nucleus and the corpus striatum.
   C.   the caudate and the thalamus.
   D.   the thalamus and the putamen
   E.   None of the above

Match the following structures with their appropriate location on the MRI:

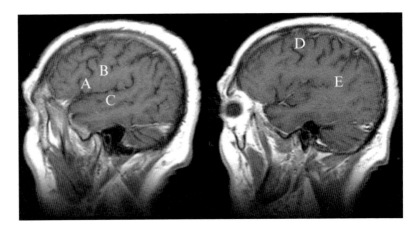

235.   Supplementary motor cortex

236.   Operculum

237.   Premotor cortex

238.   Heschl's gyrus

239.   Which of the following are true of the greater occipital nerve?
A.   It emerges inferior to the inferior obliquus capitis muscle.
B.   It is accompanied by the occipital artery.
C.   It is a sensory nerve.
D.   All of the above
E.   None of the above

240.   Which of the following statements is FALSE regarding arachidonic acid metabolism?
A.   Aspirin inhibits both cyclooxygenase (COX) isoforms.
B.   Arachidonic acid is a substrate for production of ceramide.
C.   Thromboxane synthesis inhibitors lead to depletion of arachidonic acid.
D.   Arachidonic acid is a substrate for COX I.
E.   Prostaglandin H_2PGH2 is a product of the COX enzyme.

241.   The basal ganglia output for eye movements is the
A.   subthalamic nucleus.
B.   substantia nigra pars compacta.
C.   substantia nigra pars reticulata.
D.   globus pallidus interna.
E.   globus pallidus externa.

242.   Which area receives dorsal roots?
A.   Dorsal lateral sulcus
B.   Dorsal intermediate sulcus
C.   Ventral lateral sulcus
D.   Dorsal median sulcus
E.   Ventral intermediate sulcus

243. Which statement is true in the case of a 4-year-old with the MRI scan findings shown here?

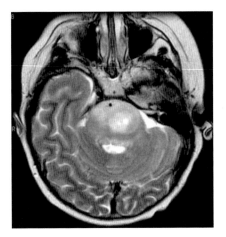

A. Biopsy is usually indicated to confirm the diagnosis.
B. Hyperfractionated radiation therapy has not been shown to improve survival.
C. It represents 30% of pediatric CNS tumors.
D. There is no proven chemotherapeutic regimen.
E. Most lesions will regress spontaneously.

244. Which of the following formulas is correct in terms of the relationship of pelvic tilt (PT), pelvic incidence (PI), and sacral slope (SS)?

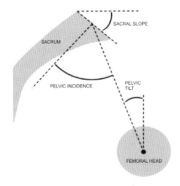

A. $PT = PI + SS$
B. $PI = PT + SS$
C. $SS = PI + PT$
D. $PT = PI - SS$
E. $SS = PI \div PT$

245.   The scan shown here was taken from a patient with a prolactin level of 267 mg/dL.

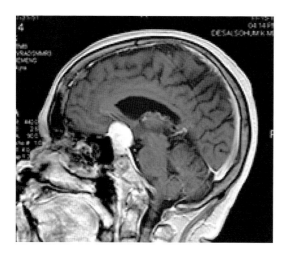

Which of the following is FALSE?
A.   Men may not seek early attention despite loss of libido and potency, headache, or fatigue.
B.   When visual loss or disturbing endocrine symptoms are present most seek medical attention.
C.   A useful endocrine test is determination of the basal serum prolactin level.
D.   The normal level ranges from 5 to 20 ng/mL.
E.   When the level of prolactin is normal post-treatment, ovulation and menstruation return in < 50% of women in galactorrhea cases.

246.   Increased prolactin is typically seen in all the following physiological states EXCEPT:
A.   Exercise
B.   Stress
C.   Sleep
D.   Pregnancy
E.   Delivery

247.   With surgical resection of the mass (shown above with Question 245), cure can be achieved in what percentage of patients?
A.   10%
B.   20%
C.   40%
D.   70%
E.   90%

248. All of the following are true of Lhermitte–Duclos disease EXCEPT:
    A. It is also called dysplastic gangliocytoma of the cerebellum.
    B. There is demyelination of granular cell layer of the cerebellum.
    C. There is thickening of one or more cerebellar folia.
    D. Calcification and hydrocephalus may occur in this disorder.
    E. A laminated pattern of folia on T2-MRI scans is suggestive of the disease.

249. Which of the following is consistent with the diagnosis of typical trigeminal neuralgia?
    A. Unilateral symptoms
    B. Sensory deficit
    C. Decreased corneal reflex
    D. All of the above
    E. None of the above

250. n-Butyl cyanoacrylate is used for
    A. cranioplasty.
    B. endovascular procedures.
    C. topical wound dressings.
    D. vasospasm in the ICU.
    E. spinal fusion.

251. A 24-year-old man is brought into the emergency room after sustaining a motorcycle accident. He has a scalp wound that is bleeding profusely. His eyes open only after his name is loudly called; however, he is confused when asked about the details of the accident. He obeys commands in all extremities. In this case, the GCS score is
    A. 15.
    B. 14.
    C. 13.
    D. 12.
    E. 11.

252. The ciliospinal center of Budge can be found at which spinal cord level?
    A. Midcervical
    B. Upper thoracic
    C. Lower thoracic
    D. Lumbar
    E. Sacral

253. The serum level of phenytoin is increased by all of the following EXCEPT:
   A.   Cimetidine
   B.   Chloramphenicol
   C.   Valproic acid
   D.   Uremia
   E.   Aspirin

254. Which of the following deficits or findings in lateral medullary syndrome is contralateral to the primary pathology?
   A.   Pain and temperature of the body
   B.   Pain and temperature of the face
   C.   Horner's syndrome
   D.   Falling
   E.   None of the above

255. Which of the following fractures is most commonly associated with anterior cord syndrome?
   A.   Clay shoveler's fracture
   B.   Wedge fracture
   C.   Teardrop fracture
   D.   Chance fracture
   E.   None of the above

256. With regard to surgical techniques on pituitary tumors, which of the following is FALSE?
   A.   Lacerations in the gland with attendant subcapsular bleeding make it difficult if not impossible to detect the subtle differences between the normal gland and a small tumor.
   B.   Prolactin microadenomas are usually situated medially in the gland.
   C.   Larger pituitary tumors usually erode the floor of the sella turcica, and in these cases the tumor may extrude into the operative wound upon removal of the floor of the sella and opening of the dura mater.
   D.   Frequently, the pituitary gland is compressed and flattened against the dorsum sellae or diaphragma sellae by tumor.
   E.   Reported incidence of postoperative CSF rhinorrhea is ~3%.

257. All of the following structures are derived from ectoderm EXCEPT:
   A.   Pia
   B.   Dura
   C.   Arachnoid
   D.   Glia
   E.   Ependyma

258. The most common primary tumor of the septum pellucidum is
    A.   meningioma.
    B.   oligodendroglioma.
    C.   astrocytoma.
    D.   ependymoma.
    E.   None of the above

259. Which of the following is the most common conflicting vessel in trigeminal neuralgia?
    A.   AICA
    B.   PICA
    C.   SCA
    D.   Satellite veins
    E.   None of the above

260. The ELANA technique may be helpful in
    A.   vertebrobasilar ischemia.
    B.   controlling ICP
    C.   vasospasm.
    D.   tumor biology.
    E.   None of the above

261. This cervical spine MRI scan demonstrates

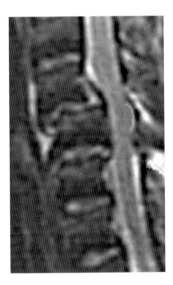

    A.   metastatic disease.
    B.   jumped facet.
    C.   burst fracture.
    D.   teardrop fracture.
    E.   epidural abscess.

262. A 64-year-old woman presents to the clinic with a left thalamic arteriovenous malformation (AVM). The lesion appears to be ~5 cm in its greatest dimension. The AVM drains exclusively to the deep venous system via several stenotic veins. How would one best grade this AVM?

A. Spetzler–Martin grade 3
B. Spetzler–Martin grade 3A
C. Spetzler–Martin grade 4
D. Spetzler–Martin grade 4A
E. Spetzler–Martin grade 5

263. Which type of breathing pattern is associated with a dorsomedial lesion in the medulla?

A. Apneustic
B. Biot
C. Central neurogenic hyperventilation
D. Kussmaul
E. Cheyne–Stokes

264. Which of the following structures is supplied mainly by the anterior choroidal artery?

A. Globus pallidus externa, posterior limb of the internal capsule
B. Globus pallidus interna, posterior limb of the internal capsule
C. Globus pallidus externa, anterior limb of the internal capsule
D. Globus pallidus interna, anterior limb of the internal capsule
E. None of the above

265. A feature that distinguishes pronator teres syndrome from carpal tunnel syndrome is that the former

A. is due to repetitive usage.
B. causes aching and fatiguing of the muscles involved.
C. causes nocturnal exacerbations.
D. exhibits numbness in the palm area.
E. is a better candidate for surgery.

266. The scan shown here was taken from a 24-year-old patient with headaches. Of the following, which is the least likely symptom or sign to manifest upon presentation?

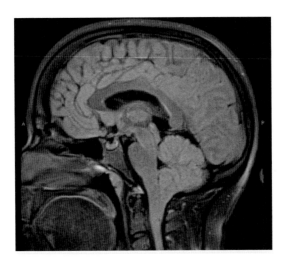

A. Weakness in the upper extremities
B. Loss of temperature sensation in lower extremities
C. Horner's sign
D. Gait disturbances
E. Diplopia

267. Which of the following is the most common reported complication in the immediate post-operative period of decompression of the lesion above?
A. Herniation of cerebellar hemispheres
B. CSF leak
C. Respiratory depression
D. Vascular injury to the posterior inferior cerebellar artery
E. Postoperative wound infection

268. Which of the following statements is FALSE regarding the lesion above?
A. Patients presenting with pain generally respond well to surgery.
B. Weakness is most likely to improve with surgery as compared with pain and sensory deficits.
C. Sensation may improve when the posterior columns are unaffected.
D. The most favorable results occurred in patients with cerebellar syndrome.
E. Factors that correlate with a worse outcome include ataxia, scoliosis, and symptoms lasting longer than 2 years.

269.   A patient states that he has a sharp electric-like pain that begins when he touches the lower side of his nose. The pain then shoots down into the cheek, then up above the eye. Which of the following divisions should be treated?
   A. V_1 only
   B. V_2 only
   C. V_3 only
   D. V_2 and V_3
   E. V_1, V_2, and V_3

270.   Gerstmann's syndrome classically includes all of the following EXCEPT:
   A.   Agraphia without alexia
   B.   Left–right confusion
   C.   Finger agnosia
   D.   Acalculia
   E.   Astereognosis

271.   A 50-year-old man is seen in clinic after being involved in a motor vehicle accident 6 months ago. He has noticed a palpable lump growing on the left side of his head (see X-ray). On examination, the lesion is painless when palpated. Which of the following lesions is most likely?

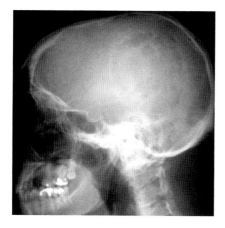

   A.   Fibrous dysplasia
   B.   Osteoma
   C.   Eosinophilic granuloma
   D.   Giant cell tumor
   E.   Epidermoid

272.   Which of the following cranial nerves exits the brainstem between the pyramid and the olive?
   A.   Cochlear
   B.   Glossopharyngeal
   C.   Vagus
   D.   Accessory
   E.   Hypoglossal

273. All of the following regarding stage 4 sleep are true EXCEPT:
    A. Dreaming occurs.
    B. Nightmares occur.
    C. There is decreased duration with hypothyroidism.
    D. Somnambulism occurs.
    E. There is increased duration after sleep deprivation.

274. Tyrosine hydroxylase is essential in the pathway for synthesizing
    A. dopamine.
    B. norepinephrine.
    C. serotonin.
    D. dopamine and norepinephrine.
    E. None of the above

275. Which of the following muscles is/are typically involved in anterior interosseous syndrome?
    A. Flexor digitorum profundus
    B. Flexor pollicis longus
    C. Pronator quadratus
    D. All of the above
    E. None of the above

276. During surgery for a petrous tumor, brisk venous bleeding is encountered at this step in the procedure (see intraoperative picture). What vascular structure is the most likely cause of this bleeding?

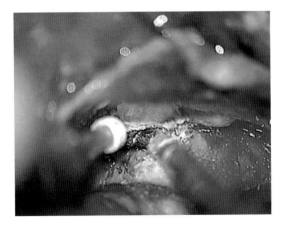

    A. Inferior petrosal sinus
    B. Jugular bulb
    C. Sigmoid sinus
    D. Transverse sinus
    E. PICA

277. Which of the following has an intact blood–brain barrier?
   A. Subforniceal organ
   B. Subcommissural organ
   C. Area postrema
   D. All of the above
   E. None of the above

278. Dysgeusia is often associated with the use of
   A. penicillin.
   B. captopril.
   C. steroids.
   D. All of the above
   E. None of the above

279. A 42-year-old man complains of a several-week history of hand numbness and clumsiness. Today he presents with severe headache and neck stiffness. What would be the best mode of treatment for the lesion depicted in the angiogram?

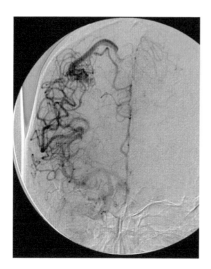

   A. Observation
   B. Surgical excision
   C. Gamma knife
   D. Partial surgical treatment
   E. Lumbar drainage

280. Which of the following is NOT associated with chronic alcoholism?
   A.   Cerebral atrophy
   B.   Wernicke's encephalopathy
   C.   Central pontine myelinolysis
   D.   Foster Kennedy's syndrome
   E.   Marchiafava–Bignami's disease

281. The patient is a 56-year-old man with mental status changes over the past several months. His wife states that he has lost his job because he was acting inappropriately. He saw a neurologist last week who conducted a single photon emission computed tomographic (SPECT) study. From the results of this study shown here, what is the cause of the dementing illness?

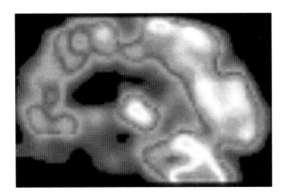

   A.   Early Alzheimer's disease
   B.   Pick's disease
   C.   Creutzfeldt–Jakob Disease
   D.   Huntington's disease
   E.   Diffuse Lewy body dementia

282. All of the following statements about fibrillation potentials are true EXCEPT:
   A.   They are a triphasic potential.
   B.   They typically last 10–15 milliseconds.
   C.   They are caused by denervation.
   D.   They are seen with poliomyelitis, ALS, and peripheral nerve injury.
   E.   They may be associated with positive sharp waves.

283. Bursts of 13 Hz lasting from half a second to 2 seconds is characteristic of
   A.   stage 1 sleep.
   B.   stage 2 sleep.
   C.   stage 3 sleep.
   D.   stage 4 sleep.
   E.   REM sleep.

284. During dissection for clipping of a large basilar artery aneurysm, a large bony protrusion is seen blocking the neck of the aneurysm (see intraoperative picture). What is this bony promontory?

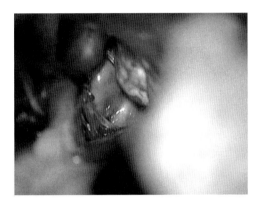

   A.   Petrous bone
   B.   Hyperostosis
   C.   Anterior clinoid process
   D.   Posterior clinoid process
   E.   None of the above

285. The transverse scapular ligament may be the cause of an entrapment syndrome which results in shoulder pain and muscle atrophy. The nerve that is trapped is
   A.   a direct branch of the C5 root.
   B.   a branch from the middle trunk.
   C.   a branch from the posterior cord.
   D.   a branch from the superior trunk.
   E.   None of the above

286. Which of the following cranial nerves travels through medial lemniscal fibers on exiting the brainstem?
   A.   III
   B.   IV
   C.   VI
   D.   VII
   E.   XII

287. Normal cerebral blood flow is
    A. 50 mL/100 mg/min.
    B. 50 mL/100 g/min.
    C. 50 mL/mg/min.
    D. 50 mL/g/min.
    E. None of the above

288. Which of the following disorders is/are associated with gustatory dysfunction?
    A. Bell's palsy
    B. Familial dysautonomia
    C. Raeder's paratrigeminal syndrome
    D. All of the above
    E. None of the above

289. Total excision of the lesion shown here is most likely to improve

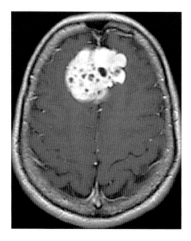

    A. attention.
    B. memory.
    C. visuoconstructive ability.
    D. executive function.
    E. cognitive function.

290. Damage to the pituitary stalk
    A. causes decreased secretion of all pituitary hormones.
    B. is independent from the hypophyseal portal system.
    C. is independent from damage to hypothalamic neurons.
    D. causes increased release of luteinizing hormone (LH).
    E. causes increased secretion of prolactin (PRL).

291. During saccadic movement of the eyes
   A.   there is increased activity of STN (subthalamic) neurons.
   B.   there is increased activity of SNpr (pars reticulata) neurons.
   C.   there is decreased activity of SNpr neurons.
   D.   there is increased activity of GPe (globus pallidus pars externa) neurons.
   E.   All of the above occur

292. All the following are true statements regarding fasciculation potentials EXCEPT:
   A.   They have three to five phases.
   B.   They last from 5 to 15 milliseconds.
   C.   They are associated with nerve fiber irritability.
   D.   They are not visible through the skin.
   E.   They may be associated with hypocalcemia, hypothermia, and nerve entrapments.

293. Calexcitin is a signaling molecule that amplifies calcium elevation in response to learning-associated synaptic transmitters in a model system of learning and memory (marine snail *Hermissenda*). Which of the following is FALSE regarding calexcitin?
   A.   Neural mechanisms regarding associative learning rarely are conserved between different species.
   B.   Calexcitin binds guanosine triphosphate (GTP), which is important in cell signaling.
   C.   At the endoplasmic reticulum membrane, it has been shown to bind to the ryanodine receptor with high affinity.
   D.   Calexcitin directly inactivates voltage-dependent potassium currents.
   E.   It is a high-affinity substrate for the α-isozyme of protein kinase C (PKC).

294. Which of the following has been described with oat cell carcinoma of the lung?
   A.   Anti-Hu antibodies and Lambert-Eaton myasthenic syndrome
   B.   Lambert-Eaton myasthenic syndrome and limbic encephalitis
   C.   Ectopic adrenocorticotropic hormone (ACTH) secretion
   D.   Syndrome of inappropriate antidiuretic hormone (SIADH)
   E.   All of the above

295. On an electrocardiogram, a J-point elevation is characteristic of
   A.   hypocalcemia.
   B.   hypokalemia.
   C.   hypothermia.
   D.   hypothyroidism.
   E.   subendocardial ischemia.

296. Which of the following encephaloceles have the greatest chance of normal intellectual development and are least likely to develop hydrocephalus?
 A. Anterior encephaloceles
 B. Parietal encephaloceles
 C. Basal encephaloceles
 D. Occipital encephaloceles
 E. Encephaloceles without nasal deformities

297. The brain tumor shown in this pathology slide expresses a high frequency of this mutation.

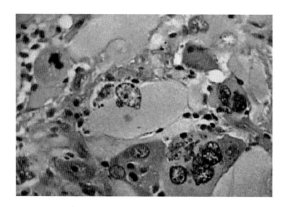

 A. TP53
 B. PTEN
 C. EGFR
 D. All of the above
 E. None of the above

298. Which of the following may be seen with anaplastic oligodendroglioma?
 A. Microvascular proliferation
 B. Necrosis
 C. Pseudopalisading
 D. All of the above
 E. None of the above

299. Which structure straddles the posterior reach of the sylvian fissure?
 A. Angular gyrus
 B. Supramarginal gyrus
 C. Middle temporal gyrus
 D. Superior parietal lobule
 E. None of the above

300.   Avellis's syndrome is most likely caused by a lesion in which area?
   A.   Medulla
   B.   Pons
   C.   Hypothalamus
   D.   Thalamus
   E.   Midbrain

301.   Bicuculline is a
   A.   glutamate agonist.
   B.   glutamate antagonist.
   C.   dopamine agonist.
   D.   GABA agonist.
   E.   GABA antagonist.

302.   All of the following statements regarding Charcot–Marie–Tooth disease are true EXCEPT:
   A.   It may be associated with a footdrop.
   B.   It is a condition of disordered myelination from decreased production of peripheral myelin protein 22 (PMP22).
   C.   It is the most common inherited peripheral neuropathy.
   D.   It is associated with a mutation on chromosome 17.
   E.   It is characterized by peroneal muscle atrophy.

303.   Neurons that give rise to the ventral trigeminothalamic tract arise from the
   A.   trigeminal motor nucleus and the spinal trigeminal tract.
   B.   dorsal aspect of the principle sensory nucleus and the spinal trigeminal tract.
   C.   ventral aspect of the principle sensory nucleus and the spinal trigeminal tract.
   D.   ventral aspect of the principle sensory nucleus and the mesencephalic tract.
   E.   dorsal aspect of the principle sensory nucleus and the mesencephalic tract.

304.   All of the following regarding motion perception are true EXCEPT:
   A.   Motion is perceived by an object's change of position on the retina.
   B.   The sensation of movement is known as the phi phenomenon.
   C.   Images that change positions more than 15 times per second are indistinguishable from continuous motion.
   D.   The motion system is disabled at rates below 100 Hz.
   E.   There is no physical process occurring on the retina that corresponds to the perceived sensation of motion.

305. Which tract decussates in the dorsal tegmental decussation?
   A. Rubrospinal tract
   B. Medial vestibulospinal tract
   C. Tectospinal tract
   D. All of the above
   E. None of the above

306. In paranasal sinus cancers, sphenoid sinus involvement is noteworthy because of which of the following?
   A. It is the major predictor of later tumor recurrence.
   B. It demands use of special instruments.
   C. It will more likely result in anosmia postoperatively.
   D. All of the above
   E. None of the above

307. Which of the following is a distinct interneuron between receptor and ganglion cell?
   A. Rods
   B. Cones
   C. Horizontal cells
   D. Amacrine cells
   E. Bipolar cells

308. Ependymoma is immunoreactive for
   A. GFAP.
   B. S-100.
   C. vimentin.
   D. All of the above
   E. None of the above

309. The caudal remnant of the median prosencephalic vein unites with the developing internal cerebral veins to form
   A. the straight sinus.
   B. the vein of Galen.
   C. the confluence of sinuses.
   D. the inferior sagittal sinus.
   E. None of the above

310. Which of the following statements is NOT true of Pelizaeus–Merzbacher disease?
   A. It has been linked to severe deficiency of myelin-specific lipids.
   B. It is X-linked recessive in the classical form.
   C. The connatal form (type II) is milder than the classical form.
   D. It manifests as a "tigroid" pattern of perivascular myelin preservation on MRI.
   E. Rare instances of female cases have been described.

311. Which afferent cerebellar tract does NOT pass through the inferior cerebellar peduncle?
  A. Reticulocerebellar
  B. Vestibulocerebellar
  C. Trigeminocerebellar
  D. Pontocerebellar tract
  E. Olivocerebellar tract

312. All of the following statements regarding the cerebellum are true EXCEPT:
  A. The flocculonodular lobe receives input from the vestibular nuclei.
  B. The anterior lobe receives input from the spinocerebellar tracts.
  C. The vermis sends fibers to the VL thalamus and motor cortex.
  D. The intermediate zone functions with posture, tone, and ipsilateral limb movements.
  E. A lesion of the interposed nuclei causes intention tremor.

313. Which of the following inhibitory synaptic connections is found exclusively in the olfactory bulb?
  A. Dendrodendritic
  B. Axodendritic
  C. Axoaxonic
  D. Axosomatic
  E. Dendroaxonic

314. Which of the following statements is FALSE regarding the parvocellular system of the lateral geniculate nucleus?
  A. It is a small cell with a compact dendritic tree.
  B. It represents a minority of the total ganglion cell number.
  C. It projects to layer $4C\beta$ in the striate cortex.
  D. It is involved with color processing.
  E. It has low contrast sensitivity and high acuity.

315. All the following are true regarding venous air embolism EXCEPT:
  A. It manifests as a decrease in end tidal CO_2.
  B. Air should be aspirated from the right atrium if it occurs.
  C. The patient should be placed in the left lateral decubitus position.
  D. The head should be lowered if possible.
  E. End tidal CO_2 changes cannot precede precordial Doppler changes.

316. The stria terminalis is a fiber tract that parallels the
  A. caudate vein.
  B. septal vein.
  C. basal vein of Rosenthal.
  D. internal cerebral vein.
  E. thalamostriate vein.

317. What are the major contents of the proximal portion of the cubital fossa, in order from medial to lateral?
   A.   Median nerve, brachial artery, biceps brachii tendon, radial nerve
   B.   Median nerve, biceps brachii tendon, radial nerve, brachial artery
   C.   Biceps brachii tendon, median nerve, radial nerve, brachial artery
   D.   Brachial artery, biceps brachii tendon, radial nerve, median nerve
   E.   None of the above

318. All of the following are medial rotators of the arm EXCEPT:
   A.   Pectoralis major
   B.   Subscapularis
   C.   Teres major
   D.   Teres minor
   E.   Latissimus dorsi

319. The medial posterior choroidal artery when viewed on an angiogram occupies the same location as this structure seen on the venous phase of the angiogram.
   A.   Vein of Galen
   B.   Basal vein of Rosenthal
   C.   Internal cerebral vein
   D.   Thalamostriate vein
   E.   Caudate vein

320. Occlusion of which of the following arteries is most likely to result in ipsilateral hypoglossal palsy?
   A.   Basilar
   B.   Anterior spinal
   C.   Vertebral
   D.   PICA
   E.   AICA

321. The Botzinger complex is a cluster of cells that are involved in
   A.   excitatory control of cardiac function.
   B.   inhibitory control of cardiac function.
   C.   excitatory control of respiratory function.
   D.   inhibitory control of respiratory function.
   E.   None of the above

322. The upper subscapular nerve arises from which segment of the brachial plexus?
   A.   Superior trunk
   B.   Medial trunk
   C.   Lateral cord
   D.   Posterior cord
   E.   Medial cord

323. All of the following are true of moyamoya disease EXCEPT:
- **A.** The majority of adults with this disease present with ischemia.
- **B.** The age of onset of symptoms displays a bimodal distribution.
- **C.** It is of unknown etiology.
- **D.** It involves progressive stenosis of the supraclinoid carotid arteries with the concomitant formation of rich collaterals at the skull base.
- **E.** It is associated with Down syndrome and neurofibromatosis.

324. All of the following are true of valproic acid EXCEPT:
- **A.** It is effective in generalized tonicoclonic seizures.
- **B.** It is ~90% protein bound.
- **C.** It has a long half-life.
- **D.** It may be associated with platelet dysfunction.
- **E.** It may result in liver dysfunction.

325. Which of the following anesthetics allows patients to emerge faster from anesthesia and has the least effect on metabolism of antiepileptic drugs?
- **A.** Enflurane
- **B.** Isoflurane
- **C.** Nitrous oxide
- **D.** Halothane
- **E.** Ketamine

326. The glomus is a prominent tuft of choroid plexus found in
- **A.** the frontal horn.
- **B.** the temporal horn.
- **C.** the atrium.
- **D.** the occipital horn.
- **E.** None of the above

327. Which of the following groups of nerves is most likely to be affected by fractures of the humerus?
- **A.** Axillary, musculocutaneous
- **B.** Median, musculocutaneous
- **C.** Axillary, radial, ulnar
- **D.** Median, radial, ulnar
- **E.** Median, radial

328. Apraxia usually results from a lesion of the
- **A.** precentral gyrus.
- **B.** postcentral gyrus.
- **C.** premotor cortex.
- **D.** prefrontal cortex.
- **E.** cingulated gyrus.

329.   On an angiogram, the colliculocentral point is halfway between tuberculum sellae and the sinus confluence. This point is closest to which structure?
  A.   Vein of Galen
  B.   Basal vein of Rosenthal
  C.   Internal cerebral vein
  D.   Straight sinus
  E.   Precentral cerebellar vein

330.   Theta activity can be described for which of the following frequencies?
  A.   5 Hz
  B.   10 Hz
  C.   15 Hz
  D.   20 Hz
  E.   25 Hz

331.   Cells of which area have true unipolar neurons?
  A.   Motor nucleus of V (trigeminal)
  B.   Mesencephalic nucleus of V
  C.   Sensory nucleus of V
  D.   Red nucleus
  E.   Locus ceruleus

332.   The spinal border cells found in the ventral horns at L1–S2 give rise to
  A.   first-order neurons of the ventral spinocerebellar tract.
  B.   second-order neurons of the ventral spinocerebellar tract.
  C.   first-order neurons of the dorsal spinocerebellar tract.
  D.   second-order neurons of the dorsal spinocerebellar tract.
  E.   None of the above

333.   Chromophobe pituitary cells
  A.   represent corticotrope cells.
  B.   stain purple after periodic acid-Schiff (PAS) staining.
  C.   represent somatotrope cells.
  D.   lack cytoplasmic granules.
  E.   can only be acidophils or basophils.

334.   Both retrospective and prospective studies of anterior temporal lobectomy have shown that seizure control in medial temporal lobe epilepsy is related to the extent of
  A.   anterior resection.
  B.   posterior resection.
  C.   lateral resection.
  D.   medial resection.
  E.   None of the above

335. Overall, the most common type of chorea is
  A. Huntington's chorea.
  B. chorea gravidarum.
  C. senile chorea.
  D. hysterical chorea.
  E. Sydenham's chorea.

336. Side effects of the medication shown here include

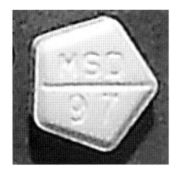

  A. myopathy.
  B. susceptibility to infection.
  C. posterior subcapsular cataracts.
  D. All of the above
  E. None of the above

337. Which of the following is true concerning relationships to the flexor retinaculum?
  A. The ulnar artery is superficial to it.
  B. The median nerve is deep to it.
  C. The ulnar nerve is superficial to it.
  D. All of the above
  E. None of the above

338. If a patient has already had a thalamotomy for tremor and now seeks treatment for tremor of the other hand, which deep brain stimulation (DBS) procedure should be done?
  A. Thalamotomy
  B. Ventralis intermedius stimulation
  C. GPi stimulation
  D. Any of the above
  E. None of the above

339. Temozolomide is a chemotherapeutic agent approved for use in treating
   A. meningioma.
   B. arteriovenous malformations.
   C. anaplastic astrocytoma.
   D. ependymomas.
   E. None of the above

340. The H-reflex is most useful to assess
   A. polyneuropathy.
   B. cervical radiculopathy.
   C. myopathy.
   D. S1 radiculopathy.
   E. median nerve compression.

341. Which of the following is NOT a normal phenomenon in the aging neuron?
   A. Lipofuscin accumulation
   B. Lewy bodies
   C. Marinesco bodies
   D. Alzheimer changes
   E. Colloid inclusions

342. A patient is asked to close his eyes during the neurological exam and the doctor places a key in the patient's hand. The ability of the patient to tell what the object is depends on the integrity of which pathway?
   A. Dorsal column
   B. Spinospinal
   C. Ventral spinocerebellar
   D. Dorsal spinocerebellar
   E. Spinothalamic

343. All of the following are true regarding intracranial pressure monitoring EXCEPT:
   A. Pressure gradients between left and right sides of the brain and supra- and infratentorial compartments may be present.
   B. The incidence of hemorrhage after insertion is about 1%.
   C. Irrigating the tubing decreases the contamination rate of ventricular catheters.
   D. Decreased intracranial compliance is suggested when the "b wavelet" is greater than the "a wavelet."
   E. There is no clear consensus as to whether to use prophylactic antibiotics.

344. Which of the following is FALSE regarding the corticospinal tract?
- **A.** In the pyramidal decussation, arm areas of cortex cross rostral to those that arise from leg areas.
- **B.** It receives contribution from somatomotor cortex, prefrontal regions, and parietal areas.
- **C.** Glutamate is present in cortical efferent fibers that project to the spinal cord.
- **D.** Leg fibers are lateral to arm fibers at most levels of this particular tract.
- **E.** Area 4 and postcentral gyrus fibers terminate in the same spinal cord lamina.

345. The middle cerebral artery supplies all of the following structures EXCEPT:
- **A.** The inferior parietal lobule
- **B.** Broca's area
- **C.** Wernicke's area
- **D.** The primary auditory cortex
- **E.** The paracentral lobule

346. During a transcallosal approach to a tumor, the risk of left hemialexia is minimized by preserving
- **A.** the genu of the corpus callosum.
- **B.** the cingulate gyrus.
- **C.** the pericallosal artery.
- **D.** the splenium of the corpus callosum.
- **E.** None of the above

347. The clivoaxial angle is normally about
- **A.** 13 degrees.
- **B.** 30 degrees.
- **C.** 100 degrees.
- **D.** 130 degrees.
- **E.** 180 degrees.

348. The sensorimotor region is located in which part of the GPi?
- **A.** Anteromedial
- **B.** Anterolateral
- **C.** Posteromedial
- **D.** Posterolateral
- **E.** None of the above

349. This lesion is resected from the lumbar spine (see intraoperative picture). Which of the following statements is FALSE?

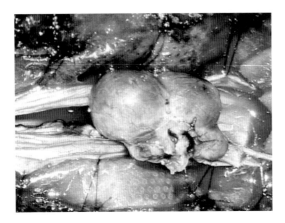

- **A.** The majority of these lesions arise from a ventral nerve root.
- **B.** 10 to 15% extend through the dural root sleeve.
- **C.** The fourth through sixth decades represent the peak incidence of occurrence.
- **D.** These masses are typically described as smooth globoid and do not produce enlargement of the nerve.
- **E.** They are suspended eccentrically from the nerve root with a discrete attachment.

350. Which of the following is particular to type I muscle fibers?
- **A.** Anaerobic
- **B.** Fast
- **C.** Stain dark with ATPase at pH 9.4
- **D.** Are found in red muscle
- **E.** Have few mitochondria

351. Which of the following pathological inclusions is intranuclear?
- **A.** Pick bodies
- **B.** Lewy bodies
- **C.** Cowdry type B bodies
- **D.** Bunina bodies
- **E.** Lafora bodies

352. All of the following tracts decussate EXCEPT:
- **A.** Lateral spinothalamic
- **B.** Ventral spinocerebellar
- **C.** Ventral corticospinal
- **D.** Dorsal spinocerebellar
- **E.** Ventral spinothalamic

353. Which of the following is most accurate of Ménière's disease?
  A.   Nystagmus is horizontal and ipsilateral to the affected side.
  B.   Nystagmus is vertical.
  C.   Falling and past-pointing are contralateral.
  D.   Nystagmus is contralateral to the affected side.
  E.   None of the above

354. Which of the following thalamic nuclei has reciprocal connections with the inferior parietal lobule?
  A.   Pulvinar
  B.   Anterior nucleus
  C.   Centromedian nucleus
  D.   VA nucleus
  E.   VL nucleus

355. Visual–verbal disconnection syndrome is most likely to be seen with sectioning of the
  A.   anterior commissure.
  B.   hippocampal commissure.
  C.   body of the corpus callosum.
  D.   genu of the corpus callosum.
  E.   splenium of the corpus callosum.

356. Pineal tumors usually displace the precentral cerebellar vein
  A.   anterosuperiorly.
  B.   posterosuperiorly.
  C.   anteroinferiorly.
  D.   posteroinferiorly.
  E.   None of the above

357. Which of the following structures can be found two-thirds of the way from the vomer to the foramen magnum?
  A.   Occipital condyle
  B.   Inion
  C.   Pharyngeal tubercle
  D.   Pituitary gland
  E.   Sphenoid sinus

358. Which of the following arteries supply the choroid plexus?
  A.   Posterior inferior cerebellar artery
  B.   Posterior cerebral artery
  C.   Anterior choroidal artery
  D.   All of the above
  E.   None of the above

359.   Which one of the following neurological manifestations is NOT associated with hepatic encephalopathy?
   A.   Asterixis
   B.   Slowing of the EEG waves
   C.   Increased levels of ammonia
   D.   Increased levels of GABA neurotransmitter
   E.   Decreased levels of glutamate

360.   Which statement regarding hepatolenticular degeneration disease is FALSE?
   A.   Serum ceruloplasmin is low.
   B.   Urinary copper is increased.
   C.   The gene locus is on chromosome 13.
   D.   Inheritance is autosomal dominant.
   E.   Early in the course of the disease, liver biopsy shows a high copper content.

361.   Which of the following is FALSE regarding Bergmann glia?
   A.   They serve as guides for migrating granular cell neurons during development.
   B.   They have cell bodies located in the molecular layer of the cerebellar cortex.
   C.   They undergo reactive gliosis adjacent to infarcts.
   D.   They extend long cytoplasmic processes through the molecular layer to the subpial surface.
   E.   They are inconspicuous until stimulated by local damage.

362.   A 62-year-old man presents with cauda equina syndrome from a herniated disk. All of the following statements are true EXCEPT:
   A.   The signs are frequently unilateral.
   B.   It classically involves spinal roots inferior to L3.
   C.   It may result in profound motor defects.
   D.   It may result in urinary or fecal incontinence.
   E.   It usually results in a Babinski sign.

363.   The vestibule contains
   A.   the kinetic labyrinth.
   B.   the ampullae.
   C.   the static labyrinth.
   D.   the cochlear duct.
   E.   None of the above

364. The ipsilateral central tegmental tract gives projections to which nucleus of the thalamus?
  A. VA
  B. VL
  C. VPL
  D. VPM
  E. None of the above

365. A meningioma located at the lateral tentorial notch with major extension infratentorially would be best managed with
  A. a lateral suboccipital retrosigmoid approach.
  B. a combined subtemporal presigmoid approach.
  C. an infratentorial supracerebellar approach.
  D. a suboccipital transtentorial approach.
  E. a pterional approach

366. Pineal calcifications are considered abnormal if encountered in patients younger than
  A. 6 years.
  B. 12 years.
  C. 18 years.
  D. 26 years.
  E. 30 years.

367. Which of the following ligaments is found between the anterior tubercle of the atlas and the dens?
  A. Anterior longitudinal ligament
  B. Posterior longitudinal ligament
  C. Alar ligament
  D. Transverse ligament
  E. None of the above

368. The most frequent site for a subependymoma is the
  A. third ventricle.
  B. fourth ventricle.
  C. left lateral ventricle.
  D. right lateral ventricle.
  E. septum pellucidum.

369. The lamina terminalis is continuous with
  A. the anterior commissure.
  B. the fornix.
  C. the rostrum of the corpus callosum.
  D. the mammillary body.
  E. None of the above

370. Damage to Brodmann area 8 on the right results in
    A. both eyes being deviated to the right at rest.
    B. both eyes being deviated to the left at rest.
    C. the right eye being "down-and-out."
    D. the patient being unable to look upward.
    E. both eyes being deviated upward.

371. Immunoreactivity to transthyretin and S-100 would most likely be seen in
    A. oligodendroglioma.
    B. low-grade astrocytoma.
    C. pleomorphic xanthoastrocytoma.
    D. choroid plexus papilloma.
    E. schwannoma.

372. Electroencephalographic (EG) activity becomes isoelectric at a cerebral blood flow of
    A. 7 mL/100 g/min.
    B. 16 mL/100 g/min.
    C. 30 mL/100 g/min.
    D. 35 mL/100 g/min.
    E. 45 mL/100 g/min.

373. All of the following are true regarding the lateral vestibulospinal tract EXCEPT:
    A. It arises from the ipsilateral Deiter's nucleus.
    B. It is located in the lateral pontine tegmentum.
    C. It crosses the midline with MLF fibers.
    D. It facilitates extensor muscle tone in the antigravity muscles.
    E. It is found at all spinal cord levels.

374. Lesions of this thalamic nucleus are found in patients with the Korsakoff amnestic state.
    A. Anterior nucleus
    B. Centromedian nucleus
    C. Pulvinar
    D. VA
    E. Mediodorsal nucleus

375. Before one transects the tentorium, which cranial nerve must be identified?
    A. III
    B. IV
    C. V
    D. VI
    E. VII

376. All the following statements regarding germ cell tumors are true EXCEPT:
- **A.** They are the most common parapineal neoplasm.
- **B.** They occur predominantly in males.
- **C.** They commonly occur at around age 30 and above.
- **D.** They are five to ten times more likely in Japan.
- **E.** They are infiltrated by T cell lymphocytes.

377. All of the following regarding CNS sarcoid are true EXCEPT:
- **A.** It is sensitive to steroids.
- **B.** It may mimic multiple sclerosis.
- **C.** It can involve cranial nerves.
- **D.** It is characterized pathologically by caseating granulomas.
- **E.** Leptomeningeal involvement is common.

378. Which of the following is the most frequent brain tumor in the first year of life?
- **A.** Choroid plexus tumor
- **B.** Gliosarcoma
- **C.** Cystic astrocytoma
- **D.** Oligodendroglioma
- **E.** Glioblastoma multiforme

379. A "square" anterior cerebral artery (ACA) shift on a cerebral angiogram suggests that there may be a mass in which area?
- **A.** Frontal lobe
- **B.** Temporal lobe
- **C.** Parietal lobe
- **D.** Occipital lobe
- **E.** Basal ganglia

380. The motor nucleus of the trigeminal nerve is located in the
- **A.** upper midbrain.
- **B.** lower midbrain.
- **C.** upper pons.
- **D.** middle pons.
- **E.** lower pons.

381. Circumventricular organs include all of the following EXCEPT:
- **A.** Obex
- **B.** Subcommissural organ
- **C.** Median eminence
- **D.** Organum vasculosum of the lamina terminalis
- **E.** Area postrema

382. Hyponatremia may be a direct cause of subarachnoid hemorrhage (SAH) from rupture of which of the following aneurysms?
- **A.** Pericallosal
- **B.** Anterior communicating
- **C.** Posterior communicating
- **D.** Middle cerebral
- **E.** Superior hypophyseal

383. All of the following are true statements of the posterior inferior cerebellar artery (PICA) EXCEPT:
- **A.** It is a branch of the vertebral artery.
- **B.** It supplies the vestibular nuclei in the medulla.
- **C.** It supplies the medial lemniscus in the medulla.
- **D.** It supplies the inferior cerebellar peduncle.
- **E.** It supplies the lateral spinothalamic tract.

384. The optic disc
- **A.** is located lateral to the fovea.
- **B.** contains myelinated axons from the retinal ganglion cell layer of the retina.
- **C.** contains only cones.
- **D.** All of the above
- **E.** None of the above

385. Which muscle is the border of the superior and inferior suboccipital triangles?
- **A.** Rectus capitis posterior major
- **B.** Superior obliquus capitis
- **C.** Inferior obliquus capitis
- **D.** Longissimus capitis
- **E.** None of the above

386. The key to translabyrinthine dissection is anatomical identification of
- **A.** the trigeminal nerve.
- **B.** the abducens nerve.
- **C.** the facial nerve.
- **D.** All of the above
- **E.** None of the above

387. All of the following are true of thoracic spine meningiomas EXCEPT:
- **A.** The great majority of spinal meningiomas occur in females.
- **B.** The most common presenting symptom is pain.
- **C.** Plain film calcification is often seen.
- **D.** Inversion recovery sequences and use of gadolinium increase detection sensitivity.
- **E.** Calcospheres may be seen.

388. Damage to the posterior cord of the brachial plexus results in paralysis of all of the following muscles EXCEPT:
  A. Teres minor
  B. Teres major
  C. Latissimus dorsi
  D. Subscapularis
  E. Infraspinatus

389. Which of the following statements is FALSE regarding radiation injury after stereotactic radiosurgery?
  A. Time of development is directly related to the rate of turnover of the cells.
  B. Cell loss after radiation occurs in connection with the cell division.
  C. Time of development is directly dependent on the radiation dose.
  D. Slowly proliferating tissue like CNS may take years to show the effects.
  E. All of the above statements are true.

390. Inherited mitochondrial disorders include all of the following EXCEPT:
  A. Leigh's disease
  B. MERFF
  C. MELAS
  D. Kearns–Sayre's syndrome
  E. Kawasaki's disease

391. Chromosomal alterations that are known to occur in tumors include all of the following EXCEPT:
  A. Loss of heterozygosity (LOH) at 1p and 19q in oligodendrogliomas
  B. LOH at 22 in ependymomas
  C. LOH at 17 in astrocytomas
  D. Monosomy of 22 in ATRT
  E. Amplification of N-myc in glioblastoma

392. During routine preoperative screening for meningioma excision, the single greatest contraindication to surgery would be
  A. myocardial infarction within the last 6 months.
  B. age greater than 75.
  C. more than five ventricular ectopic beats per minute.
  D. smoking more than one pack of cigarettes a day.
  E. being hepatitis C positive.

393. All of the following tracts pass through the inferior cerebellar peduncle EXCEPT:
  A. Dorsal spinocerebellar
  B. Cuneocerebellar
  C. Fastigiovestibular
  D. Olivocerebellar
  E. Vestibulocerebellar

394. A lower altitudinal hemianopia is the results of
  A. unilateral destruction of the cuneus.
  B. bilateral destruction of both cunei.
  C. unilateral destruction of the lingual gyrus.
  D. bilateral destruction of both lingual gyri.
  E. None of the above

395. During clipping of the unruptured aneurysm shown here, what is the best maneuver to minimize rupture?

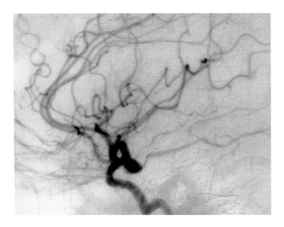

  A. Temporary clipping of the carotid in the neck
  B. Lumbar drainage
  C. Preoperative use of steroids
  D. Keeping the patient intubated until surgery
  E. Minimal retraction

396. The reasons for monitoring wave 5 during acoustic neuroma surgery include which of the following?
  A. It is an indication of the activity peripheral to the tumor.
  B. It is easier to detect than the other waves.
  C. Wave 5 is an accurate predictor of hearing postoperatively regardless of N1.
  D. All of the above
  E. None of the above

397. All of the following are true of multiple sclerosis EXCEPT:
  A. Axons are intact.
  B. Unidentified bright objects (UBOs) may be seen on MRI.
  C. Active lesions show contrast enhancement.
  D. Initial symptoms are referable to motor function.
  E. About 10 percent have a positive family history.

398.   All of the following are structures of the circuit of Papez EXCEPT:
  A.   Anterior thalamus
  B.   Cingulated gyrus
  C.   Fornix
  D.   Hippocampus
  E.   Dorsomedial thalamus

399.   Leigh's disease is a disease of the mitochondria that has an autosomal recessive inheritance. Which one of the following is not a manifestation of this metabolic disease?
  A.   White matter degeneration affecting mostly subcortical U-fibers
  B.   Bilateral spongiform degeneration of the thalamus and basal ganglia
  C.   Degeneration of the peripheral nerves
  D.   Degeneration of the spinal cord
  E.   Degeneration of the brainstem

400.   A nonfluent, expressive aphasia can result from damage to
  A.   Brodmann area 40.
  B.   Brodmann area 41.
  C.   Brodmann area 42.
  D.   Brodmann area 43.
  E.   Brodmann area 44.

401.   Levels of N-acetylaspartic acid in the urine and CSF are elevated in
  A.   adrenoleukodystrophy.
  B.   Canavan's disease.
  C.   Alexander's disease.
  D.   Krabbe's disease.
  E.   metachromatic leukodystrophy.

402.   The most commonly observed platelet dysfunction encountered in surgical patients is due to
  A.   hemophilia A.
  B.   factor V deficiency.
  C.   aspirin.
  D.   heparin.
  E.   vitamin K deficiency.

403.   All of the following are RNA viruses EXCEPT:
  A.   Poxvirus
  B.   Picornavirus
  C.   Paramyxovirus
  D.   Reovirus
  E.   Rhabdovirus

404. Hematoporphyrin derivative (HPD) is used in
    A. radiotherapy.
    B. chemotherapy.
    C. gene therapy.
    D. photochemotherapy.
    E. None of the above

405. The cranial nerve most sensitive to radiation is
    A. I.
    B. II.
    C. III.
    D. IV.
    E. V.

406. The mastoid emissary vein is a useful guide to approximate the location of
    A. the junction of the transverse and sigmoid sinuses.
    B. the jugular bulb.
    C. AICA.
    D. All of the above
    E. None of the above

407. In the spinal cord, lamina 3 and 4 are also known as
    A. the substantia gelatinosa.
    B. the nucleus proprius.
    C. the zona intermedia.
    D. All of the above
    E. None of the above

408. The cerebellar glomerulus includes all of the following EXCEPT:
    A. Mossy fibers terminal
    B. Golgi cell dendrite
    C. Granule cell dendrite
    D. Purkinje cell
    E. Golgi cell axon terminal

409. The most common histological feature detected as a late sign of radiation injury is
    A. cellular apoptosis.
    B. endothelial cell proliferation.
    C. demyelination of the nerve fibers.
    D. diffuse vasculitis.
    E. focal white matter necrosis.

410. Which spinal cord level has the most gray matter and the least white matter?
   A. Cervical
   B. Thoracic
   C. Lumbar
   D. Sacral
   E. None of the above

411. This disorder resulting from a mutation of the signaling molecule NOTCH3 on chromosome 19 leads to subcortical white matter ischemic damage.
   A. MERRF
   B. CADASIL
   C. MPS IV
   D. HHT
   E. VHL

412. The most common side effect of high-dose dexamethasone is
   A. hyperglycemia.
   B. psychosis.
   C. exacerbation of peptic ulcer.
   D. aseptic necrosis.
   E. skin rash.

413. All of the following regarding cryptococcal meningitis is true EXCEPT:
   A. Patients rarely complain of headache.
   B. Nausea, vomiting, mental status changes, and cranial nerve palsies are features.
   C. It is caused by an encapsulated budding yeast.
   D. In some communities, it is more common than toxoplasmosis as a cause of presenting neurological illness associated with HIV infection.
   E. Infection occurs by the inhalation of organisms resulting in a primary pulmonary focus of infection.

414. What percentage of cerebrospinal fluid leaks from basilar skull fractures will resolve spontaneously?
   A. 1%
   B. 15%
   C. 45%
   D. 65%
   E. 85%

415. Co-secretion of the α-subunit pituitary glycoprotein in measurable excess occurs in pituitary tumors that secrete
   A. PRL.
   B. ACTH.
   C. TSH.
   D. All of the above
   E. None of the above

416. During the caloric test, the superior vestibular nerve constitutes the main afferent from
   A.   the superior semicircular canal.
   B.   the lateral semicircular canal.
   C.   the posterior semicircular canal.
   D.   All of the above
   E.   None of the above

417. The inferior orbital fissure is mainly formed by
   A.   the sphenoid bone only.
   B.   the sphenoid and ethmoid bones.
   C.   the zygomatic and palatine bones.
   D.   the sphenoid and maxilla.
   E.   None of the above

418. Many spinocerebellar fibers are distributed to
   A.   the medial vermal region of the anterior lobe.
   B.   the lateral region of anterior lobe.
   C.   the medial vermal region of posterior lobe.
   D.   the lateral region of posterior lobe.
   E.   None of the above

419. Which of the following is NOT an indication for stereotactic radiosurgery?
   A.   Cerebral arteriovenous malformation
   B.   Metastatic tumor from non–small cell lung carcinoma
   C.   1 cm acoustic schwannoma limited to the IAC
   D.   1.5 cm petrous apex meningioma not distorting the brainstem
   E.   1 cm aneurysm at the top of basilar artery

420. All the following are true about the tumor represented by the CT scan and intraoperative picture shown here, EXCEPT:

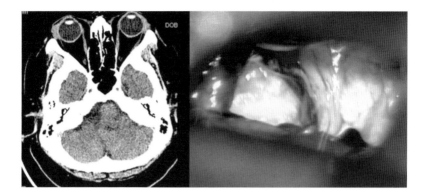

- **A.** Initial symptoms present between ages 20–40 years.
- **B.** It may cause longstanding ventriculitis.
- **C.** It is associated with midline fusion defect.
- **D.** It is characterized by linear growth.
- **E.** Spillage of tumor contents in the subarachnoid space must be avoided.

421. All of the following disorders are autosomal recessive EXCEPT:
- **A.** Maple syrup urine disease
- **B.** Adrenoleukodystrophy
- **C.** Wilson's disease
- **D.** Refsum's disease
- **E.** Homocystinuria

422. In cerebral salt wasting syndrome patients are usually
- **A.** hypervolemic and hypernatremic.
- **B.** hypervolemic and hyponatremic.
- **C.** hypovolemic and hypernatremic.
- **D.** hypovolemic and hyponatremic.
- **E.** None of the above

423. All of the following are true of toxoplasmosis EXCEPT:
- **A.** It is the most common cause of intracerebral mass associated with HIV infection when CD4 counts fall below $100/mm^3$.
- **B.** Chorea in a patient with AIDS may be pathognomonic of toxoplasmosis.
- **C.** Radiographic images show an asymmetric target sign.
- **D.** The presenting neurological symptom is nonfocal and superimposed on a global encephalopathy.
- **E.** Therapy includes pyrimethamine and sulfadiazine.

424. The fracture that initiates a leptomeningeal cyst most commonly involves the
A. frontal bone.
B. sphenoid bone.
C. temporal bone.
D. parietal bone.
E. occipital bone.

425. Which of the following medical therapies for pituitary tumors is known for its side effect of gallstone formation?
A. Bromocriptine
B. GnRH agonists
C. Octreotide
D. All of the above
E. None of the above

426. Which of the following is a reasonable criterion for recommending stereotactic surgery for acoustic neuroma?
A. The patient is elderly with a medium-sized tumor.
B. The patient has recently been hospitalized and is on two "heart medications" and a "water pill."
C. The tumor is on the side of the patient's only hearing ear.
D. All of the above
E. None of the above

427. Bill's bar is a bony protuberance that separates
A. the facial and superior vestibular nerves.
B. the facial and inferior vestibular nerves.
C. the acoustic and superior vestibular nerves.
D. the acoustic and inferior vestibular nerves.
E. None of the above

428. Which of the following persistent circulations is the most common?
A. Trigeminal artery
B. Otic artery
C. Hypoglossal artery
D. Proatlantal intersegmental artery
E. Posterior communicating artery

429. A 42-year-old professional musician presents to the neurosurgery clinic with a complaint of "blocked feeling in my ear." An axial, gadolinium-enhanced, T1-weighted MRI scan at the internal acoustic canal level is shown in the imaging. Management strategies may include all of the following EXCEPT:

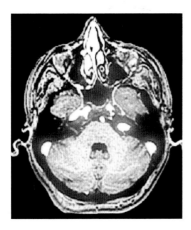

    A. Audiogram with pure tones and speech reception
    B. Counseling regarding the options of surgery or radiosurgery
    C. Workup for a planned craniotomy
    D. Consent for angiography and possible embolization
    E. Observation

430. An upper homonymous quadrantanopia is most likely to arise from a lesion to the
    A. ipsilateral parietal lobe.
    B. contralateral parietal lobe.
    C. ipsilateral temporal lobe.
    D. contralateral temporal lobe.
    E. occipital cortex.

431. All of the following neurogenetic diseases display trinucleotide repeat EXCEPT:
    A. Fragile X syndrome
    B. Myotonic dystrophy
    C. Olivopontocerebellar atrophy
    D. Huntington's disease
    E. Machado–Joseph's disease

432. An early symptom of a patient approaching local anesthetic overdose is
    A. chest tightening.
    B. lightheadedness.
    C. tingling around the mouth.
    D. shortness of breath.
    E. focal seizures.

433. Regarding motor skill learning, which of the following is most accurate of a motor act performed repeatedly and mastered?
   A. There is progressive attenuation of the cerebellar and premotor areas, but no change of activity in the primary motor cortex.
   B. There is progressive attenuation of the cerebellar, but no change in the premotor and primary motor cortices.
   C. There is no change in the cerebellar, but progressive attenuation of the premotor and primary motor cortices.
   D. There is no change in the cerebellar and premotor cortices, but progressive attenuation of the primary motor cortex.
   E. There is no change in activity of the cerebellar, premotor, or primary motor cortex.

434. All of the following are true of extradural hematomas EXCEPT:
   A. They can appear crescentic.
   B. The lucid interval is seen in ~ 80% of patients.
   C. A dry eye postoperatively can occur from traction injury of a nerve.
   D. Outcome correlates well with the clinical state prior to surgery.
   E. Outcome is inversely correlated with delay in surgery.

435. Major indications for craniotomy for pituitary tumors include
   A. tumor extension into the middle fossae.
   B. a dumbbell shape with constriction in the middle of the tumor.
   C. a tumor claimed to be fibrous on previous transsphenoidal resection.
   D. All of the above
   E. None of the above

436. An auditory brainstem implant (ABI) is most useful during tumor removal when placed in the
   A. third ventricle.
   B. jugular vein.
   C. lateral recess of the fourth ventricle.
   D. lumbar cistern.
   E. cisterna magna.

437. The nerve that innervates the rhomboids and levator scapula arises from which segment of the brachial plexus?
   A. Root
   B. Trunk
   C. Division
   D. Cord
   E. Branch

438. Which of the following conditions is associated with neurofibrillary tangles?
- **A.** Alzheimer's disease
- **B.** Down's syndrome
- **C.** Progressive supranuclear palsy
- **D.** SSPE
- **E.** All of the above

439. A patient has a subarachnoid hemorrhage from the aneurysm shown here. During surgery via right craniotomy, what part of normal brain may be removed to gain better visualization of the aneurysm?

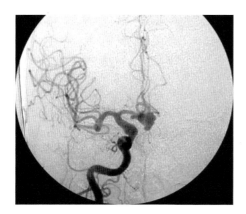

- **A.** The temporal tip
- **B.** The area lateral to cranial nerve I
- **C.** The right-sided inferior frontal gyrus
- **D.** All of the above
- **E.** None of the above

440. The ophthalmic artery pierces the dura to enter the orbit near the
- **A.** anterior clinoid process.
- **B.** oculomotor nerve.
- **C.** optic strut.
- **D.** trochlear nerve.
- **E.** vomer.

441. The cuneus lies between which sulci?
- **A.** Sulcus cinguli and parieto-occipital sulcus
- **B.** Calcarine and cingulate
- **C.** Sylvian and calcarine
- **D.** Parieto-occipital and calcarine
- **E.** None of the above

442.   Regarding cerebral aneurysms which of the following statements is FALSE?
  A.   Oxyhemoglobin and bilirubin are the agents likely producing the meningeal response.
  B.   The size of an intracerebral hematoma is directly related to the chance of the patient developing vasospasm.
  C.   Only ~ 1% of cerebral aneurysms result in subdural bleeding.
  D.   A cerebral aneurysm has a single layer of endothelium.
  E.   The most important factor in assessing bleeding risk is the temporal relationship to the previous bleed.

443.   Volatile anesthetics
  A.   reduce cerebral metabolic rate (CMR) and increase cerebral blood flow (CBF).
  B.   reduce CMR and CBF.
  C.   increase CMR and CBF.
  D.   increase CMR and reduce CBF.
  E.   have no effect on CMR and increase CBF.

444.   Prolonged ulnar and median F response latencies could represent a conduction block in the
  A.   upper trunk.
  B.   upper and middle trunk.
  C.   middle trunk.
  D.   roots of C5 and C6.
  E.   lower trunk.

445.   An abnormal skin histamine response is a characteristic feature of
  A.   Horner's syndrome.
  B.   Frey's syndrome.
  C.   Chagas's disease.
  D.   Familial dysautonomia.
  E.   Huntington's disease.

446.   Which foramen of the cranial base is situated at the junction of the occipital and temporal bone?
  A.   Foramen ovale
  B.   Foramen magnum
  C.   Jugular foramen
  D.   All of the above
  E.   None of the above

447.   Which tract is a projection from the habenulum?
  A.   Diagonal band of Broca
  B.   Fasciculus retroflexus
  C.   Ansa lenticularis
  D.   Lenticular fasciculus
  E.   Obex

448. Which of the following is true of microaneurysms?
- **A.** They form as part of normal aging but are not affected by hypertension.
- **B.** They form as part of normal aging and are accentuated by hypertension.
- **C.** They are not part of the normal aging process and are not affected by hypertension.
- **D.** They are not part of normal aging and are accentuated by hypertension.
- **E.** They usually affect blood vessels > 300 µm in diameter.

449. Contrast-enhanced axial T1-weighted MRI scans of a 56-year-old man are shown in this image. The most likely symptoms he might have are

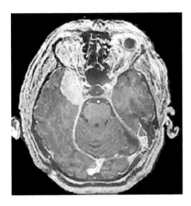

- **A.** dizziness, ataxia, and balance problems.
- **B.** expressive aphasia with positive Rhomberg's sign.
- **C.** tinnitus and reduced hearing in the right ear with frequent falling.
- **D.** ptosis of the right eye with weakness of external ocular muscles.
- **E.** weakness in the right side of body, especially in the upper limbs.

450. Which artery is most closely associated with cranial nerves VII and VIII?
- **A.** Superior cerebellar artery
- **B.** Basilar artery
- **C.** AICA
- **D.** PICA
- **E.** Vertebral artery

451. The medulla includes all of the following structures EXCEPT:
- **A.** Olive
- **B.** Tuberculum cinereum
- **C.** Vagal trigone
- **D.** Facial colliculus
- **E.** Origin of the glossopharyngeal nerve

452. Regarding vascular malformations which of the following statements is FALSE?
  A. Arteriovenous malformations can contain neural parenchyma.
  B. Calcification is common in cavernous malformations.
  C. Hemosiderin-laden macrophages are common in venous malformations.
  D. Capillary malformations do not show progressive growth.
  E. Early angiographic filling is seen with AVMs

453. In a patient with subarachnoid hemorrhage, the most accurate statement regarding calcium channel blocking agents is that they have a
  A. clear beneficial effect, improve angiographic vasospasm, and increase CBF.
  B. clear beneficial effect and improve angiographic vasospasm and functional outcome.
  C. modest beneficial effect.
  D. detrimental effect.
  E. detrimental effect and decrease CBF.

454. The anatomy of the posterior inferior cerebellar artery (PICA) is such that important branches to the deep cerebellar nuclei leave the vessel at the top of the cranial loop. The name of this point and the segment of PICA it arises from are
  A. the plexal point, tonsillomedullary segment.
  B. the choroidal point, tonsillomedullary segment.
  C. the plexal point, telovelotonsillar segment.
  D. the choroidal point, telovelotonsillar segment.
  E. None of the above

455. The principal neuroanatomical substrate of perceptual organization is
  A. the anterior right hemisphere.
  B. the posterior right hemisphere.
  C. the anterior left hemisphere.
  D. the posterior left hemisphere.
  E. None of the above

456. The sigmoid sinus and the superior petrosal sinuses are boundaries of
  A. Trautmann's triangle.
  B. Parkinson's triangle.
  C. Wernicke's triangle.
  D. Labbé's triangle.
  E. Calot's triangle.

457. The lateral lemnisci are connected by
  A. the trapezoid body.
  B. the commissure of Probst.
  C. the juxtarestiform body.
  D. All of the above
  E. None of the above

458. A solid, contrast-enhancing mass of the anterior third ventricle that stains intensely for GFAP is most likely a
  A. choroid plexus tumor.
  B. colloid cyst.
  C. central neurocytoma.
  D. chordoid glioma.
  E. glioblastoma multiforme.

459. Which of the following is a contradiction of stereotactic radiosurgery in the management of metastatic tumors?
  A. Three tumors, each measuring 1–1.5 cm within the right hemisphere
  B. A solitary left parietal tumor measuring 2cm × 2cm × 1.8cm
  C. A 2.5 cm left mesial temporal tumor with clinical signs of herniation
  D. Tumors in both the supratentorial and the infratentorial compartment
  E. No tissue biopsy from the brain

460. The sphenoparietal sinus can be found at the
  A. outer aspect of the lesser wing of the sphenoid.
  B. inner aspect of the lesser wing of the sphenoid.
  C. outer aspect of the greater wing of the sphenoid.
  D. inner aspect of the greater wing of the sphenoid.
  E. cavernous sinus.

461. The precuneus (area 7) can be found
  A. on the lateral aspect of the frontal lobe.
  B. on the medial aspect of the frontal lobe.
  C. on the lateral aspect of the occipital lobe.
  D. on the medial aspect of the occipital lobe.
  E. on the medial aspect of the parietal lobe.

462. The most common cerebral vascular malformation is
  A. capillary telangiectasia.
  B. venous malformation.
  C. arteriovenous malformation.
  D. cavernous malformation.
  E. dural arteriovenous fistula.

463. The anterior meningeal artery typically arises from the
  A. ophthalmic artery.
  B. maxillary artery.
  C. middle meningeal artery.
  D. occipital artery.
  E. facial artery.

464.   The caudal anterior limb of the internal capsule is supplied by
    A.   the middle cerebral artery.
    B.   the internal cerebral artery.
    C.   the recurrent artery of Heubner.
    D.   the posterior communicating artery.
    E.   None of the above

465.   The external urethral sphincter is composed mainly of _____ fibers arranged in a _____ fashion.
    A.   type I, longitudinal
    B.   type II, longitudinal
    C.   type I, circular
    D.   type II, circular
    E.   None of the above

466.   Regarding atlanto-occipital dislocation all of the following are true EXCEPT:
    A.   It should be suspected in a multitrauma victim with mandibular fractures and submental lacerations.
    B.   Prevertebral soft tissue swelling may be the only clue to its diagnosis.
    C.   The gap between the occipital condyles and condylar surface of the atlas is >5 mm.
    D.   The distance between the tip of the dens and the basion is <12 mm.
    E.   The clivus line is not tangential to the odontoid.

467.   The action potential in the neuron is initiated at the
    A.   dendrite.
    B.   soma.
    C.   hillock.
    D.   node of Ranvier.
    E.   axon terminal.

468.   Which of the following conditions is most often associated with chronic temporal lobe epilepsy?
    A.   Pilocytic astrocytoma
    B.   Ganglioglioma
    C.   DNET
    D.   Astrocytoma
    E.   Pleomorphic xanthoastrocytoma

469. Which of the following is not a functional indication for stereotactic radiosurgery?
   A.   Trigeminal neuralgia refractory to medication
   B.   Glossopharyngeal neuralgia in a patient with carbamazepine hypersensitivity
   C.   Unilateral essential tremors refractory to medication
   D.   Parkinson's tremor in the left upper extremity with levodopa-induced dyskinesias
   E.   Huntington's chorea

470. Regarding the venous drainage of the insula, which of the following statements is true?
   A.   The entire insula drains to the deep venous system.
   B.   The entire insula drains to the superficial venous system.
   C.   The anterior portion of the insula drains to the deep system.
   D.   The posterior portion of the insula drains to the superficial system.
   E.   None of the above

471. Which of the following separates the anterior cerebellar lobe from the posterior cerebellar lobe?
   A.   Posterolateral fissure
   B.   Horizontal fissure
   C.   Dorsolateral fissure
   D.   Primary fissure
   E.   Postlunate fissure

472. Regarding spinal vascular malformations, which of the following is FALSE?
   A.   Dural arteriovenous fistulas are believed to be acquired.
   B.   Normal neural parenchyma is seen within juvenile AVMs.
   C.   Glomus AVMs may have associated aneurysms.
   D.   Acute progression is most likely due to venous congestion.
   E.   Dural AV fistulas have a female predilection.

473. The ischemic penumbra has a cerebral blood flow of
   A.   1–8 mL/100 g/min.
   B.   8–23 mL/100 g/min.
   C.   23–30 mL/100 g/min.
   D.   30–40 mL/100 g/min.
   E.   40–50 mL/100 g/min.

474. What is the area interposed between the lenticular fasciculus and the thalamic fasciculus?
   A.   Substantia nigra
   B.   Pedunculopontine nucleus
   C.   Zona incerta
   D.   Subthalamic nucleus
   E.   None of the above

475. Which of the following areas modulate control of micturition?
   A. Medial parts of the frontal lobes
   B. Preoptic region of the hypothalamus
   C. Basal ganglia
   D. All of the above
   E. None of the above

476. The juxtarestiform body is _____ to the _____ cerebellar peduncle.
   A. Lateral, inferior
   B. Lateral, superior
   C. Medial, inferior
   D. Medial, superior
   E. None of the above

477. The flower-spray ending is associated with which nerve type?
   A. IA
   B. IB
   C. II
   D. III
   E. IV

478. When performing a caudalis rhizotomy, which tract is penetrated to access the target?
   A. Ventral spinocerebellar tract
   B. Dorsal spinocerebellar tract
   C. Gracile fasciculus
   D. Cuneate fasciculus
   E. None of the above

479. The arterial dicrotic notch
   A. has no corresponding area in the intracranial pressure (ICP) waveform.
   B. corresponds to the area between P1 and P2 of the ICP waveform.
   C. corresponds to the area between P2 and P3 of the ICP waveform.
   D. corresponds to the area after P3 of the ICP waveform.
   E. None of the above

480. The basal vein of Rosenthal begins at this area on the base of the brain.
   A. Anterior perforated substance
   B. Posterior perforated substance
   C. Tuber cinereum
   D. Medial geniculate body
   E. Lateral geniculate body

481. The calcified glomus of the choroid plexus seen on CT scan is most often found in the
   A.   frontal horn.
   B.   third ventricle.
   C.   trigone of lateral third ventricle.
   D.   occipital horn.
   E.   foramen of Monro.

482. Decussation of the superior cerebellar peduncles occurs in which area of the brain?
   A.   Cerebellum
   B.   Rostral midbrain
   C.   Rostral pons
   D.   Caudal midbrain
   E.   Caudal pons

483. Cranial nerves IX, X, and XI are supplied by the
   A.   superior thyroid artery.
   B.   ascending pharyngeal artery.
   C.   lingual artery.
   D.   facial artery.
   E.   occipital artery.

484. Attempted lateral gaze where there is destruction of the abducens nucleus results in
   A.   ipsilateral lateral and medial rectus palsies.
   B.   ipsilateral lateral and contralateral medial rectus palsies.
   C.   contralateral lateral and ipsilateral medial rectus palsies.
   D.   contralateral lateral and medial rectus palsies.
   E.   None of the above

485. Brainstem auditory evoked responses (AER) are most useful to monitor the function of
   A.   the medial lemniscus.
   B.   the lateral lemniscus.
   C.   the corticospinal tracts.
   D.   All of the above
   E.   None of the above

486. The lateral subnucleus of cranial nerve III innervates the
   A.   the inferior rectus.
   B.   the inferior oblique.
   C.   the medial rectus.
   D.   All of the above
   E.   None of the above

487.   Deep pressure and joint position is localized to
   A.   Brodmann area 3a.
   B.   Brodmann area 3b.
   C.   Brodmann area 2.
   D.   Brodmann area 1.
   E.   None of the above

488.   Which of the following is the least consistent feature of conus syndrome?
   A.   Symmetric involvement
   B.   Pain
   C.   Saddle anesthesia
   D.   Bladder and bowel symptoms
   E.   Sudden onset

489.   Malignant peripheral nerve sheath tumors (MPNSTs) most commonly affect cranial nerve
   A.   III.
   B.   IV.
   C.   V.
   D.   VI.
   E.   VII.

490.   The superior ophthalmic vein courses most closely with which cranial nerves?
   A.   IV (trochlear) and V (trigeminal)
   B.   III (oculomotor) and IV
   C.   III and II (optic)
   D.   V and VI (abducens)
   E.   II and IV

491.   The caudate nucleus forms
   A.   the medial wall of the frontal horn.
   B.   the floor of the temporal horn.
   C.   the lateral wall of the occipital horn.
   D.   the roof of the lateral ventricle.
   E.   None of the above

492.   Which of the following is true regarding the dorsal trigeminothalamic tract?
   A.   It arises from the principal sensory nucleus of V.
   B.   It terminates on the VPM thalamus.
   C.   It conveys touch and pressure information from the face.
   D.   It is an uncrossed tract.
   E.   All of the above

493. Valveless emissary veins are found in which layer of the scalp?
   A. Skin
   B. Subcutaneous tissue
   C. Galea
   D. Loose areolar tissue
   E. Periosteum

494. Apocrine sweat glands in the axilla are innervated by what type of fibers?
   A. Adrenergic fibers
   B. Cholinergic fibers
   C. Nitric Oxide
   D. VIP
   E. None of the above

495. The greatest decline in water content of the nucleus pulposus occurs when?
   A. Just after birth
   B. Childhood
   C. Adolescence
   D. Young adulthood
   E. Late adulthood

496. The tapetum are fibers from
   A. the claustrum.
   B. the globus pallidus.
   C. the corpus callosum.
   D. the thalamus.
   E. None of the above

497. Dressing apraxia is most often described with lesions of the
   A. dominant frontal lobe.
   B. nondominant frontal lobe.
   C. dominant parietal lobe.
   D. nondominant parietal lobe.
   E. occipital lobe.

498. Cerebrospinal fluid is reabsorbed into the bloodstream through the
   A. valveless arachnoid villi.
   B. pressure-insensitive valves of the arachnoid villi.
   C. pressure-sensitive one-way valves of the arachnoid villi.
   D. pressure-insensitive valveless arachnoid villi.
   E. cranial nerves.

499. The precursor of ACTH is
    A. CLIP.
    B. beta-lipotropin.
    C. alpha-MSH.
    D. POMC.
    E. p53.

500. Regarding myasthenia gravis (MG), which of the following statements is FALSE?
    A. It involves autoantibodies directed against acetylcholine receptors at the neuromuscular junction,
    B. The prevalence is between 1 in 10,000 to 15,000.
    C. Juvenile MG is more common in Asians.
    D. There is an increased incidence of an underlying thymoma in late-onset MG.
    E. Late-onset MG is more common in females.

501. The internal carotid artery (ICA) enters the cranium via a canal formed by the
    A. sphenoid bone.
    B. occipital bone.
    C. sphenoid and temporal bones.
    D. temporal bone.
    E. temporal and occipital bones.

502. All of the following are true of the trochlear nerve EXCEPT:
    A. It has a nucleus located in the midbrain tegmentum at the level of the inferior colliculus.
    B. It decussates in the superior medullary velum.
    C. It exits the brainstem from the dorsal surface of the brainstem.
    D. It courses lateral to the frenulum of the superior medullary velum.
    E. Damage to the nucleus results in dysfunction of the superior oblique muscle on that side.

503. The asterion is located at the intersection of
    A. the lambdoid, occipitomastoid, and parietomastoid sutures.
    B. the lambdoid, sagittal, and occipitomastoid sutures.
    C. the lambdoid, sagittal and parietomastoid sutures.
    D. the sagittal and occipitomastoid sutures.
    E. None of the above

504. Which nucleus of the hypothalamus is involved with the dissipation of heat?
    A. Posterior nucleus
    B. Ventromedial nucleus
    C. Lateral nucleus
    D. Anterior nucleus
    E. None of the above

505. Which of the following joints lacks an intervertebral disk?
A. Occipitoatlantal joint
B. Atlantoaxial joint
C. Sacrum
D. All of the above
E. None of the above

506. The diagnosis of syndrome of inappropriate antidiuretic hormone (SIADH) is made by the following observations EXCEPT:
A. Serum sodium < 135 mEq/L
B. Serum osmolarity < 280 mOsm/L
C. Hypervolemia
D. Urine sodium > 20 mmol/24 h
E. Urine osmolarity > serum osmolarity

507. Which of the following congenital conditions results in a deficit in abduction of the eye resulting from failure of development of motor neurons in the sixth nerve nucleus?
A. Gunn's syndrome
B. Joubert's syndrome
C. De Morsier's syndrome
D. Duane's syndrome
E. None of the above

508. Dilantin levels are increased by all of the following EXCEPT:
A. Cimetidine
B. Coumadin
C. Carbamazepine
D. Isoniazid
E. Sulfa drugs

509. Which of the following fiber tracts end as climbing fibers?
A. Olivocerebellar
B. Reticulocerebellar
C. Pontocerebellar
D. All of the above
E. None of the above

510. The most relevant factor in assessing prognosis of paraganglioma patients is
A. tumor location.
B. tumor size.
C. time to surgery.
D. chemotherapy and radiation.
E. None of the above

511.   The anteromedial triangle of the middle fossa is defined by cranial nerves
   A.   IV and V_1.
   B. V_1 and V_2.
   C. V_2 and V_3.
   D. V_3 and VI.
   E.   None of the above

512.   Hyperperfusion encephalopathy most commonly involves which part of the brain?
   A.   Subcortical white matter of the occipital lobes bilaterally with little to no edema
   B.   Subcortical white matter of the occipital lobes bilaterally with edema
   C.   The cortical ribbon of the parietal lobes bilaterally
   D.   The cortical ribbon and subcortical white matter bilaterally
   E.   The cortical ribbon with sparing of the subcortical U-fibers

513.   Glasscock's triangle is defined by the posterior border of V_3 and which foramina?
   A.   Foramen ovale and spinosum
   B.   Foramen ovale and rotundum
   C.   Foramen rotundum and spinosum
   D.   Foramen spinosum and lacerum
   E.   Foramen lacerum and ovale

514.   Which of the following is FALSE regarding hyperperfusion encephalopathy?
   A.   The vast majority of patients recover completely.
   B.   The edema tends to resorb completely.
   C.   The vertebrobasilar system is vulnerable due to extensive sympathetic innervation.
   D.   A similar condition may occur after a carotid endarterectomy.
   E.   Patients with hyperperfusion encephalopathies often have labile blood pressures.

515.   All of the following are correct statements about the central sulcus EXCEPT:
   A.   It separates the frontal lobe from the parietal lobe.
   B.   It separates the motor cortex from the sensory cortex.
   C.   It extends into the paracentral lobule.
   D.   It is usually continuous with the lateral sulcus.
   E.   It is located on the lateral convex surface of the hemisphere.

516.   Which of the following is NOT a feature of migraine headaches?
   A.   Normal intraocular pressure
   B.   Ipsilateral flushing
   C.   Decreased local skin temperature
   D.   Female predominance
   E.   No aura is seen with common migraines

517. Cortical paralysis of visual fixation, optic ataxia, and disturbance of visual attention, with preservation of spontaneous and reflex eye movements, may be seen after bilateral parieto-occipital lesions. The syndrome described is
   A.   Anton's syndrome.
   B.   Adie's syndrome.
   C.   Cogan's syndrome.
   D.   Vernet's syndrome.
   E.   Balint's syndrome.

518. During a selective amygdalohippocampectomy for intractable seizures, the surgeon must be aware that the most medial part of the amygdala is in close proximity to
   A.   the basal ganglia.
   B.   the anterior commissure.
   C.   the caudate nucleus.
   D.   All of the above
   E.   None of the above

519. The anterior choroidal artery usually runs _____ to the posterior communicating artery, and _____ to the optic tract.
   A.   Lateral, parallel
   B.   Medial, parallel
   C.   Lateral, perpendicular
   D.   Medial, perpendicular
   E.   None of the above

520. Which of the following muscles is a medial rotator of the thigh?
   A.   Piriformis
   B.   Obturator internus
   C.   Quadratus femoris
   D.   Gluteus minimus
   E.   Gluteus maximus

521. Lewy bodies may be seen in all the following EXCEPT:
   A.   Parkinson's disease
   B.   Shy–Drager's syndrome
   C.   Multiple system atrophy
   D.   Diffuse Lewy body dementia
   E.   Paralysis agitans

522. The largest contributor to the internal cerebral vein is the
   A.   septal vein.
   B.   thalamostriate vein.
   C.   caudate vein.
   D.   basal vein of Rosenthal.
   E.   vein of Galen.

523. During a thalamotomy for Parkinsonian tremor, the patient reports that he has paresthesias of the fingertips and the mouth. This would most likely be due to the electrode being too
  A.   anterior to the target.
  B.   posterior to the target.
  C.   medial to the target.
  D.   lateral to the target.
  E.   close to the target.

524. Deficiencies of complement components C5–C9 predispose to
  A.   *Streptococcus pneumoniae.*
  B.   *Haemophilus influenzae.*
  C.   *Neisseria meningitidis.*
  D.   *Proteus.*
  E.   None of the above

525. Meningiomas of the ventricular system are most frequently located at the
  A.   body.
  B.   trigone.
  C.   temporal horn.
  D.   occipital horn.
  E.   frontal horn.

526. In patients with multiple cerebral metastases, the most important determinant of survival is
  A.   the size of the largest metastasis.
  B.   the extent of systemic disease.
  C.   the number of visible metastases on MRI scan.
  D.   the neurological condition preoperatively.
  E.   proximity to the eloquent cortex.

527. Sensory axons that transmit information from the Golgi tendon organs are
  A.   Ia (A-α).
  B.   Ib (A-α).
  C.   II (A-β).
  D.   III (A-δ).
  E.   IV (C).

528. The vast majority of spinal epidural abscesses can be best described as
  A.   caused by staphylococci; occur in the cervical cord.
  B.   caused by streptococci; occur in the cervical cord.
  C.   caused by staphylococci; occur in the thoracic cord.
  D.   caused by streptococci; occur in the thoracic cord.
  E.   caused by staphylococci; occur in the lumbar cord.

529. With regard to shunt infections, which of the following is FALSE?
   A. *Staphylococcus* is the organism implicated in a majority of cases.
   B. Symptoms include shunt failure, headache, nausea, and vomiting.
   C. Elevated temperature is a more reliable sign of infection in VA as opposed to VP shunts.
   D. There is a greater risk of shunt infection with distal revision than with proximal revision.
   E. *Staphylococcus* infections may cause obstruction without fever.

530. Which of the following is the most common type of tumor arising in the sella following irradiation for pituitary adenoma?
   A. Liposarcoma
   B. Fibrosarcoma
   C. Angiosarcoma
   D. Chondrosarcoma
   E. Osteosarcoma

531. Dopamine loss in Parkinson's disease is believed to lead to
   A. disinhibition of the subthalamic nucleus.
   B. high activity of Gpi/SNr.
   C. inhibition of the motor thalamus.
   D. All of the above
   E. None of the above

532. Which of the following is true regarding the etiology of postoperative diabetes insipidus?
   A. It is due to disruption of the pituitary stalk.
   B. There is degeneration of distal axons in the region of dissection.
   C. Stored ADH is depleted.
   D. All of the above
   E. None of the above

533. Which of the following parasites present with cord compression in infected patients?
   A. Strongyloides
   B. Schistosomiasis
   C. Paragonimiasis
   D. Neurocysticercosis
   E. Echinococcus

534. The mediodorsal nucleus of the thalamus is reciprocally connected to the
   A. cingulated gyrus.
   B. prefrontal cortex.
   C. substantia nigra.
   D. lateral lemniscus.
   E. inferior parietal lobule.

535. Lymphoma metastatic to the brain tends to localize to the
- **A.** subependyma.
- **B.** gray–white junction.
- **C.** meninges.
- **D.** frontal lobe.
- **E.** corpus callosum.

536. In developing an interforniceal plane for resection of an anterior third ventricular tumor, the surgeon must be most cognizant of what structure in the posterior component of the forniceal structure?
- **A.** Anterior commissure
- **B.** Posterior commissure
- **C.** Hippocampal commissure
- **D.** All of the above
- **E.** None of the above

537. All the following are true of the centromedian nucleus of the thalamus EXCEPT:
- **A.** It is the largest of the intralaminar nuclei.
- **B.** It receives input from the globus pallidus.
- **C.** It projects to the striatum.
- **D.** It projects diffusely to the entire neocortex.
- **E.** It is reciprocally connected to areas 41 and 42.

538. The stylomastoid foramen is located _____ to the insertion of the _____ belly of the digastric muscle.
- **A.** Medial, anterior
- **B.** Medial, posterior
- **C.** Lateral, anterior
- **D.** Lateral, posterior
- **E.** None of the above

539. Mutism following transcallosal surgery may be the result of
- **A.** division of the anterior corpus callosum.
- **B.** retraction on the fornix.
- **C.** circulatory disturbance in the SMA.
- **D.** All of the above
- **E.** None of the above

540. Which of the following are sources of input to the red nucleus?
- **A.** Dentate nucleus
- **B.** Globose nucleus
- **C.** Emboliform nucleus
- **D.** All of the above
- **E.** None of the above

541. Which of the following is a noncompetitive α blocker?
A.   Phentolamine
B.   Atropine
C.   Phenylephrine
D.   Amphetamine
E.   Phenoxybenzamine

542. All of the following are true regarding the cerebral metabolic rate ($CMRO_2$) EXCEPT:
A.   Forty percent of the energy consumed is for maintenance of ionic gradients.
B.   Once EEG silence is induced, barbiturates will not produce further reductions in ($CMRO_2$).
C.   Once EEG silence is induced, temperature reduction does produce further reductions in ($CMRO_2$).
D.   The normal rate is ~5 mL/100 g brain/min.
E.   Ketamine anesthesia decreases $CMRO_2$.

543. The globus pallidus projects to which thalamic nuclei?
A.   Centromedian
B.   Ventral anterior
C.   Ventral lateral
D.   All of the above
E.   None of the above

544. The major blood supply to this tumor (see image) is from the

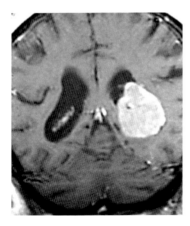

A.   posterior cerebral artery.
B.   posterior choroidal artery.
C.   middle cerebral artery.
D.   anterior choroidal artery.
E.   occipital artery.

545. Preoperative testing for this tumor (see image) should include which of the following?

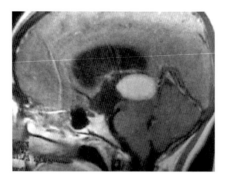

    A. α-fetoprotein
    B. β-HCG
    C. CBC, PT, PTT
    D. All of the above
    E. None of the above

546. The most medial fibers in the crus cerebri are
    A. frontopontine.
    B. corticobulbar.
    C. corticospinal.
    D. parietopontine.
    E. sympathetic fibers.

547. A 45-year-old woman is brought into the urgent care center after being involved in a motor vehicle accident while driving home with her husband. Her husband was ejected from the car from the force of the impact and did not survive. On initial examination her eyes open to pain, and she mumbles only sounds. She localizes on the right arm, withdraws on the left side, and the right leg is not examined due to the possibility of a fracture. The GCS score for this case is
    A. 11.
    B. 10.
    C. 9.
    D. 8.
    E. 7.

For questions 548 to 550, match this MRI scan with the most likely diagnosis:
    A. Glioblastoma multiforme
    B. Hemangiopericytoma
    C. Ewing's sarcoma
    D. Sinonasal carcinoma metastases
    E. Breast carcinoma metastases

548.

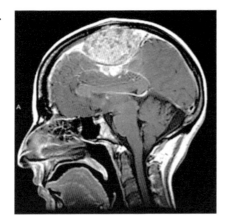

549.

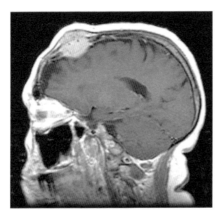

550.

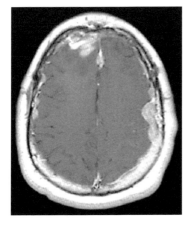

551.   Relative contraindications for surgery for spinal metastasis include all of the following EXCEPT:
   A.   Multiple myeloma
   B.   Recurrence after maximal radiation
   C.   Multiple lesions at multiple levels
   D.   Total paralysis for > 48 hours
   E.   Expected survival < 3 months

552.   Which of the following is the usual radiation dose for spinal epidural metastasis?
   A.   20 Gy in 2 Gy fractions over 10 days
   B.   30 Gy in 3 Gy fractions over 10 days
   C.   60 Gy in 6 Gy fractions over 10 days
   D.   100 Gy in 10 Gy fractions over 10 days
   E.   200 Gy in 50 Gy fractions over 30 days

Match the following toxins with the appropriate findings:
   A.   Tetanus
   B.   Botulism
   C.   Diphtheria
   D.   Reye's syndrome

553.   There is a predilection to sensory and motor nerves of the limbs and ciliary muscle/nerve.

554.   It typically presents with risus sardonicus.

555.   The initial symptom is usually difficulty in convergence of the eyes.

556.   Encephalopathy typically develops 4 to 7 days after the onset of the illness

557.   Which statement is true regarding the presentation of multiple myeloma in the spine?
   A.   Hypocalcemia occurs in 25% of patients.
   B.   Bone pain is characteristically at rest and with movement.
   C.   There is occurrence of amyloidosis.
   D.   Invasion of the spinal canal occurs in over 50% of patients.
   E.   Definitive diagnosis can be made by plain X-ray.

558.   Criteria for the diagnosis of multiple myeloma include all of the following EXCEPT:
   A.   Biopsy-proven plasmacytoma
   B.   Myeloma cells in a single peripheral blood smear
   C.   Plasma cells > 10 of 1000 cells on marrow morphology
   D.   Radiographic survey demonstrating lytic lesions
   E.   Monoclonal immunoglobulins in the urine or blood

559. The Batson plexus route of spinal metastases spread represents which type of spread?
   A. Perinervous
   B. Arterial
   C. Venous
   D. Direct extension
   E. All of the above

Match the following chromosomal abnormality with the appropriate disease or syndrome:
   A. 5q
   B. 5p
   C. 4
   D. 9
   E. None of the above

560. Facioscapulohumeral dystrophy (Landouzy–Dejerine's syndrome)

561. Werdnig–Hoffmann's disease

562. Myotonic muscular dystrophy

563. Cri du chat syndrome

564. Friedreich's ataxia

Match the antiarrhythmic with the appropriate statement:
   A. Verapamil
   B. Diltiazem
   C. Digoxin
   D. Procainamide
   E. Esmolol

565. Preferred agent for patients with systolic heart failure

566. Side effects of hypotension and negative inotropic effect

567. Indicated for chronic rate control of atrial fibrillation

568. Contraindicated in patients with prolonged QT interval

569. Indicated for rate control of atrial fibrillation in the setting of a hyperadrenergic state

570. A 56-year-old woman just had a large frontal tumor resected that stained positive for reticulin on immunostaining. The tumor histology contained mitotic figures as well as necrosis and pseudopalisading. The most likely diagnosis is
    A. ganglioglioma.
    B. gliosarcoma.
    C. glioblastoma multiforme.
    D. gliomatosis cerebri.
    E. germinoma.

571. Which of the following is true regarding management of the blunt injury shown here?

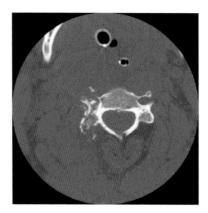

    A. Those with mild neurological deficits and accessible lesions are better managed by repair than ligation.
    B. Proximal occlusion may be accomplished by an anterior approach with mobilization of the sternocleidomastoid.
    C. Endovascular embolization with detachable balloons may be used for management.
    D. All of the above are true.
    E. None of the above are true.

Match the following metals with the corresponding syndrome:
    A. Mercury
    B. Manganese
    C. Arsenic
    D. Aluminum
    E. Lead

572. Peripheral neuropathy, malaise, nausea, and vomiting

573. Encephalitis in children

574.   Rigidity, bradykinesia

575.   Irritability, seizures, ataxia, coma

576.   Peripheral neuropathy, ataxia, renal tubular necrosis

577.   Mimics the deficit of cortical cholinergic neurotransmission seen in Alzheimer's

578.   Out of the following choices, which represents the most common source of arterial embolus?
   A.   Left atrium
   B.   Left ventricle
   C.   Pulmonary veins
   D.   Aorta
   E.   Ventricular aneurysms

579.   Potassium depletion would MOST likely result from which of the following diseases?
   A.   Diabetic ketoacidosis
   B.   Cushing's syndrome
   C.   High intestinal obstruction
   D.   Chronic diarrhea
   E.   Uremia

580.   Which of the following is the first sign of hypomagnesemia?
   A.   Seizures
   B.   Tetany
   C.   Hypotension
   D.   Loss of deep tendon reflexes
   E.   Stupor

581.   All of the following are appropriate concentrations of ions in Ringer's lactate solution EXCEPT:
   A. Na^+ 130 mEq/L
   B. Cl^- 109 mEq/L
   C.   Lactate 28 mEq/L
   D. Ca^{2+} 16 mEq/L
   E. K^+ 4 mEq/L

582. All of the following statements are associated with the type of tumor exemplified by this MRI scan EXCEPT:

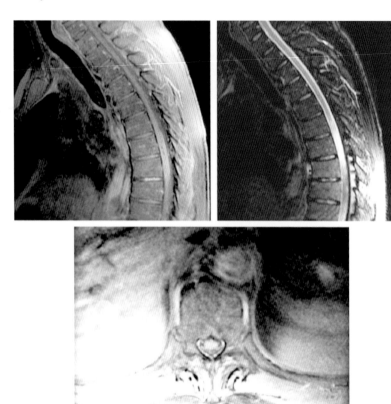

A. The male to female ratio is 1.5:1.
B. Thoracic location is the most common.
C. It is usually low grade.
D. It is the most common intramedullary tumor in children.
E. Examination may reveal a combination of upper and lower motor neuron signs.

Match the disorder with the appropriate disease:
A. Amyotrophic lateral sclerosis
B. Systemic lupus erythematosus
C. Metachromatic leukodystrophy
D. Lesch–Nyhan syndrome
E. Niemann–Pick disease

583. Arylsulfatase A deficiency

584.   Superoxide dismutase mutation

585.   HGPRT deficiency

Match the appropriate serum levels with the corresponding disease:
   A.   Increased calcium, normal phosphate, and increased alkaline phosphatase
   B.   Decreased calcium, increased phosphate, and normal alkaline phosphatase
   C.   Decreased calcium, decreased phosphate, and increased alkaline phosphatase
   D.   Normal calcium, normal phosphate, and increased alkaline phosphatase

586.   Rickets

587.   Paget's disease

588.   Hyperparathyroidism

589.   Primary osteoporosis

590.   Hypoparathyroidism

Match the blood gas and electrolyte data to the relevant acid–base disorder:
   A.   Chronic respiratory acidosis
   B.   Non-anion gap metabolic acidosis and respiratory alkalosis
   C.   Metabolic alkalosis and respiratory acidosis
   D.   Wide anion gap metabolic acidosis
   E.   Chronic respiratory alkalosis

591.   pH 7.44, pCO_2 32 mm Hg, pO_2 90 mm Hg; serum sodium 140 mEq/L; potassium 4.2 mEq/L; chloride 109 mEq/L; bicarbonate 21 mEq/L

592.   pH 7.40, pCO_2 19 mm Hg, pO_2 89 mm Hg; serum sodium, 140 mEq/L; potassium 4.3 mEq/L; chloride 117 mEq/L; bicarbonate 11 mEq/L

593.   pH 7.40, pCO_2 51 mm Hg, pO_2 87 mm Hg; serum sodium, 140 mEq/L; potassium 4.5 mEq/L; chloride 97 mEq/L; bicarbonate 31 mEq/L

594.   pH 7.32, pCO_2 50 mm Hg, pO_2 63 mm Hg; serum sodium 140 mEq/L; potassium 4 mEq/L; chloride 100 mEq/L; bicarbonate, 28 mm Hg

595.   pH 7.29, pCO$_2$ 20 mm Hg, pO$_2$ 87 mm Hg; serum sodium, 137 mEq/L; potassium 4.5 mEq/L; chloride 100 mEq/L; bicarbonate, 9 mEq/L

Match the appropriate scan with the syndrome:

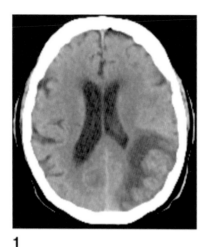

1

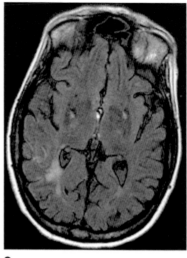

2

    A.   Scan 1
    B.   Scan 2
    C.   Scans 1 and 2
    D.   None of the above

596.   Valve prosthesis

597.   Man-in-the-barrel syndrome

598.   Perforating branch occlusion

599.   The nucleus secreting hormones that stimulate release of luteinizing hormone (LH) and follicle-stimulating hormone (FSH) and which projects to the medial eminence is
    A.   the tuberoinfundibular nucleus.
    B.   the preoptic nucleus.
    C.   the paraventricular nucleus.
    D.   the mammillary bodies.
    E.   None of the above

600. Efferent pupillary defects are seen in the following disorders EXCEPT:
  A. Adie's pupil
  B. Posterior communicating artery aneurysm
  C. Kennedy syndrome
  D. Horner's syndrome
  E. Third nerve lesion

601. Relative afferent pupillary defects are seen in the following disorders EXCEPT:
  A. Macular degeneration
  B. Optic neuritis
  C. Papilledema
  D. Metabolic optic neuropathy
  E. Retinal lesion

602. Hypoxemia due to a 50% shunt is most likely to be improved by which of the following measures?
  A. Decreasing the positive end expiratory pressure to 0 cm H_2O
  B. Hyperventilation
  C. Improving mixed venous oxygen contents
  D. Oxygen supplementation
  E. None of the above

603. The half-life of platelets used for transfusion is
  A. 96 hours.
  B. 72 hours.
  C. 48 hours.
  D. 24 hours.
  E. 12 hours.

604. Which phase of blood coagulation is the most time consuming?
  A. Conversion of prothrombin to thrombin
  B. Activation of contact factors
  C. Generation of thromboplastin
  D. Release of phospholipids from platelets
  E. Conversion of fibrinogen to fibrin

Match the appropriate scan with the these statements:

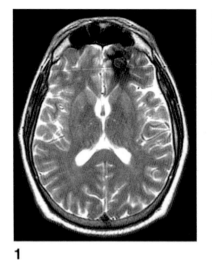

1

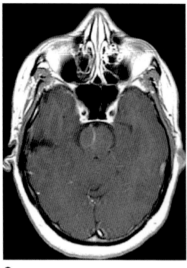

2

    A.   Image 1
    B.   Image 2
    C.   Images 1 and 2
    D.   None of the above

605.   Caused by arrested development

606.   Acquired after dural thrombosis

607.   Associated with blue rubber nevus syndrome

Match the associated ocular finding with the correct pathological state:
    A.   Ocular bobbing
    B.   Jerk nystagmus
    C.   See-saw nystagmus
    D.   Downbeat nystagmus
    E.   None of the above

608.   Foramen magnum compression

609.   Craniopharyngioma

610.   Germinoma

611.   Pentobarbital infusion

612.   Pontine glioma

Match the cerebellar cell type with the appropriate description:
  A.   Granule cell
  B.   Golgi cell
  C.   Purkinje cell
  D.   Basket cell
  E.   Stellate cell

613.   Forms the glomerulus together with the granule cell

614.   Excitatory neurotransmitter

615.   End in a rete of terminals around the cell bodies of the Purkinje cell

616.   Synapse with the interposed nuclei

617.   Which of the following is the earliest sign of cyanide poisoning?
  A.   Blurred vision
  B.   Diaphoresis
  C.   Apnea
  D.   Hallucinations
  E.   Sneezing

618.   Which of the following minerals is important in wound healing?
  A.   Manganese
  B.   Zinc
  C.   Iron
  D.   Copper
  E.   All of the above

619.   The mechanism of action of aminoglycosides is best described by
  A.   inhibition of DNA synthesis.
  B.   cell membrane destruction.
  C.   cell wall damage.
  D.   inhibition of protein synthesis.
  E.   None of the above

620. Antimicrobial agents causing neuromuscular blockade include all of the following EXCEPT:
   A. Streptomycin
   B. Kanamycin
   C. Neomycin
   D. Polymyxin
   E. Gentamicin

621. Given the aneurysm exposed by a far lateral approach (cerebellum retracted) (see intraoperative picture), which statement is true?

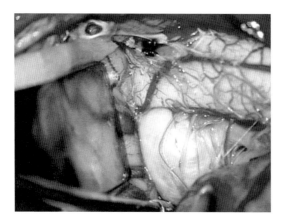

   A. The Allcock test is useful.
   B. External ventricular drainage following subarachnoid hemorrhage from this type of aneurysm is an accepted temporizing treatment.
   C. Proximal ligation is the preferred treatment.
   D. Vasospasm in this area is unlikely to cause respiratory compromise.
   E. A lumbar drain is contraindicated in this case.

622. In this tumor resection case (see intraoperative picture), which of these statements is FALSE?

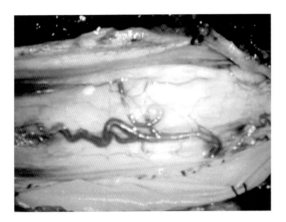

   A. The dura needs to be opened at either end well above the lesion.
   B. Dilated veins are more likely to be encountered at the rostral end of the mass.
   C. Myelotomy is to be done as close to the midline as possible.
   D. Intracapsular decompression of the tumor is necessary to avoid any traction.
   E. C-arm guidance for localization may be helpful.

623. Accumulations seen in metachromatic leukodystrophy are
   A. sulfatides.
   B. galactocerebroside.
   C. ganglioside.
   D. long-chain fatty acids.
   E. None of the above

624. The T-reflex represents
   A. flexor response as seen in decerebrate rigidity.
   B. crossed extensor reflex.
   C. monosynaptic stretch reflex.
   D. supramaximal stimulation of a mixed motor-sensory nerve.
   E. All of the above

625. The trochlear nerve arises from the brainstem at the level of the
   A. lower pons.
   B. upper pons.
   C. lower midbrain.
   D. upper midbrain.
   E. medulla.

626. A 57-year-old man with a known history of lung cancer presents with generalized muscle weakness. The most likely associated finding is
A.   opsoclonus.
B.   increased glutamic acid decarboxylase.
C.   anti–Purkinje cell antibodies.
D.   presynaptic acetylcholine receptor disorder.
E.   multiple sclerosis.

627. To produce 1 mEq/L rise in serum potassium, the total body potassium stores need to increase by what quantity?
A.   50 mEq
B.   150 mEq
C.   350 mEq
D.   500 mEq
E.   1000 mEq

628. If the C6 nerve root is severed, all of the following may be affected EXCEPT:
A.   Lateral cord
B.   Ulnar nerve
C.   Musculocutaneous nerve
D.   Median nerve
E.   Lower subscapular nerve

Match each plexus with its innervation:
A.   Brachial plexus
B.   Cervical plexus
C.   Lumbar plexus
D.   Cervical and brachial plexuses
E.   None of the above

629.   Inferior belly of the omohyoid

630.   C5 nerve root

631.   Obturator nerve

632.   Levator scapulae

633.   External urethral sphincter

634.   Sternocleidomastoid

635. Which of the following is a characteristic of narcolepsy?
   A. Hallucinations while sleeping
   B. Convulsions while sleeping
   C. Daytime hyperalertness
   D. NREM onset of sleep
   E. Gelastic seizures

For the following items, match the vitamin excess or deficiency and the clinical disorder:
   A. Thiamine
   B. B6
   C. Cobalamine
   D. Niacin
   E. Vitamin A

636. Pseudotumor cerebri

637. Beriberi

638. Increased serum homocysteine

639. Lower extremities paresthesias

Match the effect with the pharmacological agent:
   A. Type A GABA agonist
   B. Type B GABA agonist
   C. GABA antagonist
   D. No effect on GABA receptors

640. Barbiturates

641. Picrotoxin

642. Baclofen

643. Bicuculline

644. The two aneurysms seen in this intraoperative picture are

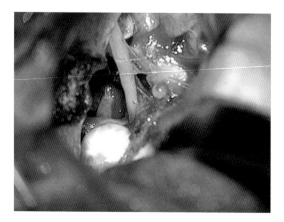

    A. anterior communicating and superior hypophyseal.
    B. basilar and anterior communicating.
    C. PICA and superior hypophyseal.
    D. PICA and basilar.
    E. basilar and posterior communicating.

645. Transcallosal approach for tumor resection shows this lesion (see intraoperative picture; the pertinent MRI is also shown). Which of the following statements is FALSE?

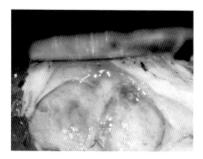 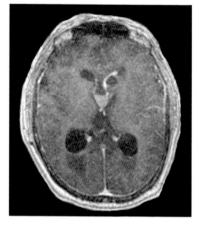

    A. A common presenting sign is papilledema.
    B. It arises from the diencephalic recess of the postvellar arch.
    C. Risk of sudden death is attributable to CSF dynamics or disturbances in hypothalamic-related cardiovascular control.
    D. Lumbar puncture is part of the initial workup.
    E. The patient may require a shunt postoperatively.

646. All of the following are associated with torsades de pointes EXCEPT:
    A. Phasic changes of amplitude and polarity of ventricular complexes
    B. Hypokalemia
    C. Hypomagnesemia
    D. Narrowed QT intervals
    E. May be predisposed by erythromycin

647. Which of the following enables one to distinguish early acute respiratory distress syndrome (ARDS) from early cardiogenic pulmonary edema?
    A. In early ARDS, the hypoxemia is more pronounced and the chest X-ray abnormalities are more evident.
    B. In early ARDS, the hypoxemia is less pronounced and the chest X-ray abnormalities are more evident.
    C. In early ARDS, the hypoxemia is more pronounced and the chest X-ray abnormalities are less evident.
    D. In early ARDS, the hypoxemia is less pronounced and the chest X-ray abnormalities are less evident.
    E. None of the above

648. All of the following are recommended therapeutic measures for diabetic ketoacidosis EXCEPT:
    A. Insulin
    B. Alkali therapy
    C. Potassium
    D. Crystalloids
    E. Phosphate

649.   A 54-year-old man who is a heavy smoker presents with balance problems and the MRI scan and pathology slide from surgery shown here. The most likely diagnosis is

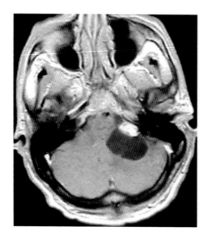 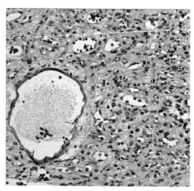

A.   metastasis.
B.   hemangioblastoma.
C.   glioma.
D.   central nervous system (CNS) lymphoma.
E.   pilocytic astrocytoma.

650. A 64-year-old man was admitted with mental status changes and a temperature of 103.4°F. Spinal fluid was obtained and showed 118 WBC, 49 RBC, 102 protein, and 79 glucose. The patient had an MRI scan, shown here. The most likely diagnosis is

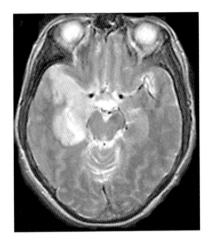

    A. glioblastoma multiforme resection.
    B. radiation therapy.
    C. trauma.
    D. encephalitis.
    E. cerebral atrophy.

651. After a motorcycle accident, a patient is able to dorsiflex and invert his foot but is unable to evert his foot. The most likely nerve lesioned is the
    A. deep peroneal nerve.
    B. superficial peroneal nerve.
    C. common peroneal nerve.
    D. sciatic nerve.
    E. tibial nerve.

652. The brachial plexus structure just distal to the division is
    A. the trunk.
    B. the branch.
    C. the cord.
    D. the root.
    E. None of the above

653. This intraoperative picture shows a middle cerebral artery bifurcation aneurysm. What is the proper order of steps to ensure safe clipping of this aneurysm?

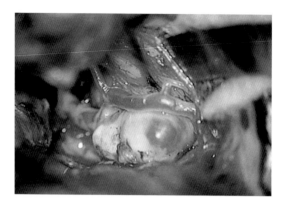

A. Definitive clipping, temporary clipping, fissure splitting, dissection of M2 branch from dome
B. Dissection of M2 branch from dome, fissure splitting, temporary clipping, definitive clipping
C. Fissure splitting, temporary clipping, dissection of M2 branch from dome, definitive clipping
D. Temporary clipping, fissure splitting, dissection of M2 branch from dome, definitive clipping
E. Fissure splitting, dissection of M2 branch from dome, temporary clipping, definitive clipping

654. Molecular genetic alterations in glioma not part of a specific syndrome include all of the following EXCEPT:
A. Overexpression of CDK4
B. Deletion of p53
C. Mutation of retinoblastoma
D. Amplification of K-ras
E. Overexpression of CDK6

655. Oligodendrogliomas exhibit loss of chromosomal regions on all the following EXCEPT:
A. 1p
B. 7
C. 9p
D. 19q
E. 22

656. All the following statements are true about the sympathetic nervous system EXCEPT:

A. Stellate ganglionectomy is used in the treatment of long QT syndrome.

B. Anhydrosis occurs with ganglionectomy.

C. Each intercostal nerve is connected to the sympathetic trunk by at least one white ramus and two gray rami.

D. The inferior hypogastric plexus lies in front of the promontory of the sacrum between the two common iliac arteries and is sometimes called the presacral nerve.

E. Sympathetically conveyed stimulus to the sweat glands is transmitted by acetylcholine.

Match the following limbic structures with the comments:

A. Cingulate gyrus

B. Hippocampus

C. Amygdala

D. Mammillary bodies

E. Anterior nucleus of the thalamus

657. Not part of the Papez circuit

658. Receives inputs from the nucleus of the solitary tract

659. Receives inputs from the medial septal nucleus

660. Which of the following has the highest incidence of associated platelet disorders?

A. Amyotrophic lateral sclerosis (ALS)

B. Huntington's disease

C. Acute respiratory distress syndrome

D. AIDS

E. Multiple sclerosis

661.   Which of the following is NOT associated with the finding on this scan?

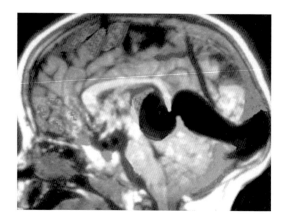

A.   Congestive heart failure
B.   Pulmonary hypertension
C.   Renal failure
D.   Microcephaly
E.   Subarachnoid hemorrhage

662.   All the following are associated with the finding on this MRI scan EXCEPT:

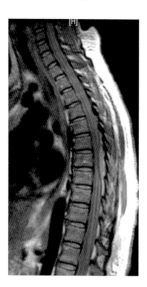

A.   The most common location is cervicothoracic.
B.   The presence of a malignancy is a predisposing condition.
C.   There is increased incidence with epidural anesthesia.
D.   The incidence is 1:10,000 in the United States.
E.   There is increased incidence with drug abuse.

663. The leading cause of magnesium deficiency is
   A. antibiotic therapy.
   B. diuretics.
   C. secretory diarrhea.
   D. diabetes mellitus.
   E. dilantin therapy.

Match the appropriate ganglion with the nerve:
   A. Jugular
   B. Nodose
   C. Pterygopalatine
   D. Ciliary
   E. Superior cervical

664. Facial nerve

665. Oculomotor nerve

666. Arnold's nerve

667. Deep petrosal nerve

668. All of the following may be used to differentiate between a lesion of the glossopharyngeal nerve and a lesion of the facial nerve EXCEPT:
   A. Loss of sensation to the outer ear
   B. Loss of taste on the tongue surface
   C. Loss of salivatory secretion from a gland
   D. Weakness of the pharynx
   E. Strength of facial muscles

669. The inotropic drug of choice for acute management of systolic heart failure is
   A. dopamine.
   B. dobutamine.
   C. neosinephrine.
   D. epinephrine.
   E. isoproterenol.

670. The toxicity of nitroprusside in the setting of decreased renal blood flow is mediated by
   A. cyanide.
   B. thiocyanate.
   C. nitric oxide.
   D. thiosulfate.
   E. vitamin B12.

Match the lesions shown here with the correct disease:

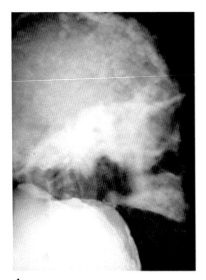

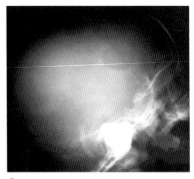

1

2

A. Lesion 1
B. Lesion 2
C. Lesions 1 and 2
D. None of the above

671. Eosinophilic granuloma

672. Langerhans cell histiocytosis

673. Paget's disease

674. Albright's syndrome

675. Epidermoid

676. The most common cause of admission of HIV-infected patients to the intensive care unit is
A. *Pneumocystis carinii* pneumonia.
B. cytomegalovirus infections.
C. toxoplasmosis.
D. AIDS encephalitis.
E. hydrocephalus.

677. An isolated exposure of broken skin or mucous membranes to HIV-infected blood carries a risk of transmission of
   A.   9%.
   B.   0.9%.
   C.   0.09%.
   D.   0.009%.
   E.   0.0009%.

678. Differential diagnosis of the lesion shown here includes the listed choices EXCEPT:

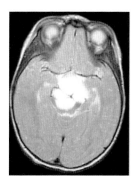 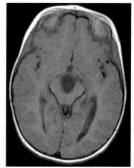

   A.   Chordoma
   B.   Epidermoid
   C.   Basilar tip aneurysm
   D.   Arachnoid cyst
   E.   Low-grade glioma

Match the appropriate organelle with its function:
   A.   Golgi organelle
   B.   Endoplasmic reticulum
   C.   Both A and B
   D.   None of the above

679. Functional ribosomes occur on the outside of its membrane but not on the inside.

680. Phosphorylation of oligosaccharides

681. Important in drug detoxification

682. Glycogen formation and breakdown

683. Lamellar or tube-like membranous system

684. Neuromelanin has the following characteristics EXCEPT:
- **A.** Accumulates in neurons of the substantia nigra
- **B.** Found in the locus ceruleus
- **C.** Made by tyrosinase
- **D.** Is a cathecholamine waste product
- **E.** Chelates metal ions such as aluminum and iron

685. Amygdala afferents include all the following EXCEPT:
- **A.** Nucleus accumbens
- **B.** Pyriform cortex
- **C.** Solitary tract nucleus
- **D.** Locus ceruleus
- **E.** Prefrontal cortex

686. All the following are complications of total parenteral nutrition EXCEPT:
- **A.** Hypercapnia
- **B.** Acalculous cholecystitis
- **C.** Impaired oxygenation
- **D.** Calculous cholecystitis
- **E.** Increased incidence of infection

687. Which of the following findings is most closely associated with the lesion on this scan?

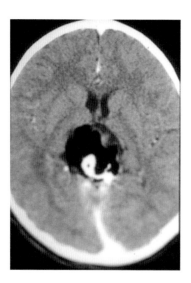

- **A.** May have elevated carcinoembryonic antigen (CEA) levels
- **B.** Associated with Schiller–Duval bodies
- **C.** Derived from extraembryonic tissue
- **D.** Ingestion of food with fecal contamination
- **E.** Multiple sclerosis

688.   Which of the following is this scan finding associated with?

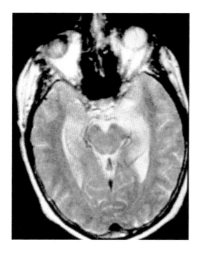

    A.   Anti-Yo antibodies
    B.   Anti-Hu antibodies
    C.   Anti-Ri antibodies
    D.   Antibodies to presynaptic voltage-gated receptors
    E.   None of the above

689.   Match the finding on this myelin-stained section with the most likely associated presentation:

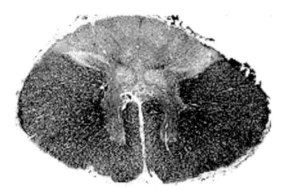

    A.   40-year-old man with chronic encephalitis and Argyll Robertson pupils
    B.   15-year-old hyperglycemic with severe lower extremity weakness
    C.   55-year-old man with spastic gait, weakness, and fasciculation in all extremities
    D.   4-year-old boy with bilateral symmetric proximal limb weakness
    E.   60-year-old female with spondylolisthesis at L5–S1

Match the following disorders with the acid–base abnormality:
- **A.**   Respiratory acidosis
- **B.**   Respiratory alkalosis
- **C.**   Both
- **D.**   Neither

690.   Pulmonary embolism

691.   Meningitis

692.   Liver cirrhosis

693.   Aminoglycosides

694.   All of the following statements are correct regarding this diffusion tractography scan EXCEPT:

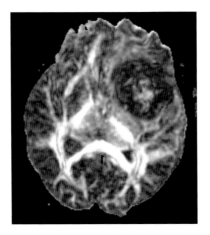

- **A.**   Water diffusion is hindered antĕriorly by the presence of a large tumor.
- **B.**   Connections between frontal and occipital lobe are impaired on the right side.
- **C.**   There are intersecting white matter tracts between the splenium and the fronto-occipital tracts.
- **D.**   Tractography gives information about the direction of flow.
- **E.**   Bundles of axons provide a barrier to perpendicular diffusion and a path for parallel diffusion along the orientation of the fibers.

695.   Which of the following is true regarding the finding on this MRI scan?

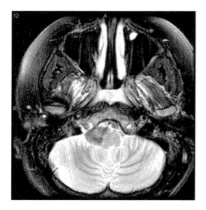 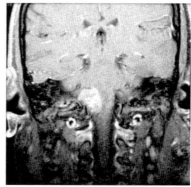

   A.   It is associated with dermal sinus tract.
   B.   It secretes histamine.
   C.   On histopathology, one may see densely packed elongated spindle cells in interlocking fascicles with a tendency toward palisading.
   D.   All of the above are true.
   E.   None of the above are true.

696.   All of the following findings may be associated with this MRI scan EXCEPT:

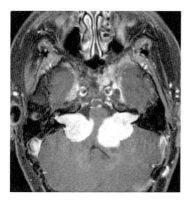

   A.   Abnormality in protein merlin
   B.   Posterior capsular lens opacities
   C.   Intertriginous freckling
   D.   Pigmented area of skin with excess hair
   E.   May be associated with an autosomal disorder located on chromosome 22

697. Etiologies of distal renal tubular acidosis include all of the following EXCEPT:
  A. Amphotericin B
  B. Lithium
  C. Toluene
  D. Carbonic anhydrase inhibitors
  E. Cyclamate

698. Which of the following is NOT a valid therapeutic measure in patients with Addisonian crisis?
  A. Hydrocortisone sodium succinate (Solucortef) for glucocorticoid emergencies
  B. Fludrocortisone (Florinef) for mineralocorticoid emergencies
  C. Methylprednisolone (Solumedrol) for glucocorticoid emergencies
  D. Cortisone acetate for glucocorticoid emergencies
  E. Intravenous fluids

699. Therapeutic measures for syndrome of inappropriate antidiuretic hormone secretion include
  A. furosemide.
  B. phenytoin.
  C. lithium.
  D. All of the above
  E. None of the above

700. Which compatible plasma types can be given to a patient with blood type B?
  A. B and O plasma types
  B. B and AB plasma types
  C. B plasma type only
  D. All of the above
  E. None of the above

701. Neurogenic shock is characterized by which of the following?
  A. Increased arteriolar tone
  B. Increased in peripheral vascular resistance
  C. Cool molten skin
  D. Hypertension
  E. Bradycardia

702. Gram-negative septicemia in hospitalized patients is MOST likely to originate from
  A. urinary tract infection.
  B. pneumonia.
  C. wound infection.
  D. gastrointestinal infection.
  E. pressure ulcers.

703. Which of the following tests has the highest sensitivity in diagnosing *Clostridium difficile* colitis?
   A.   Latex agglutination test
   B.   Tissue culture assay for cytotoxin
   C.   Stool culture
   D.   Stool microscopy
   E.   Polymerase chain reaction (PCR) analysis

Match the anesthetic with the corresponding property:
   A.   Isoflurane
   B.   Enflurane
   C.   Thiopental
   D.   Halothane

704. Increases cerebral blood flow the most

705. Decreases intracranial pressure

706. Causes transient tachycardia in children

707. Increases systemic vascular resistance

Match the finding with appropriate syndromes:
   A.   Neurofibromatosis type 1 (NF1)
   B.   Neurofibromatosis type 2 (NF2)
   C.   Both A and B
   D.   None of the above

708. Autosomal dominant inheritance

709. Retinal hemangioma

710. Iris hamartoma

711. Segmental and confined to one part of the body

712. This is an intraoperative picture showing clipping of an ophthalmic artery aneurysm. With regard to the neck of the aneurysm, which statement is true?

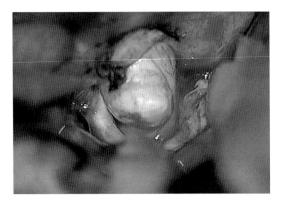

    A. The neck of the aneurysm is unobstructed.
    B. The neck of the aneurysm is obstructed by the dome.
    C. The neck of the aneurysm is obstructed by the optic nerve.
    D. The neck of the aneurysm is obstructed by the carotid artery.
    E. The neck of the aneurysm is obstructed by the anterior clinoid process.

713. During microvascular decompression for trigeminal neuralgia, this intraoperative picture is taken and the offending artery is seen. What is the artery and what structure does it come close to more proximally in this picture?

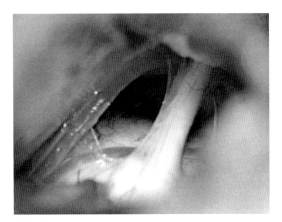

    A. Superior cerebellar artery, abducens nerve
    B. Anterior inferior cerebellar artery, trochlear nerve
    C. Superior cerebellar artery, trochlear nerve
    D. Anterior inferior cerebellar artery, abducens nerve
    E. Superior cerebellar artery, oculomotor nerve

714. Which of the following is the LEAST favorable therapeutic approach for the lesion depicted on the MRI scans?

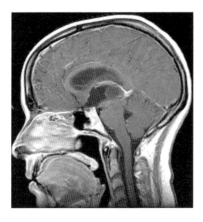 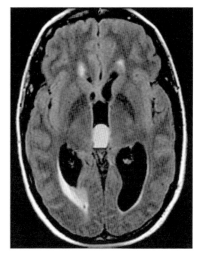

    A. Supracerebellar infratentorial approach for cyst resection
    B. Midline frontal approach for cyst resection
    C. Third ventriculostomy
    D. Midline frontal approach for cyst decompression
    E. Endoscopic cyst resection

Match the correct medication with its effect:
    A. Meperidine
    B. Thyroid hormones
    C. Fluconazole
    D. Papaverine

715. Inhibits antiparkinsonism effect of levodopa

716. Increases serum phenytoin levels

717. Enhances clotting factor catabolism

718. Decreases warfarin metabolism

719. May cause hypertension, rigidity, and excitation when used with monoamine oxidase inhibitors

720. Which of the following medications is safe to use in a patient with history of malignant hyperthermia?
   A.   Epinephrine
   B.   Isoflurane
   C.   Halothane
   D.   Thiopental
   E.   All of the above

721. Which of the following neoplasms is LEAST likely to metastasize to the spine?
   A.   Lung carcinoma
   B.   Breast carcinoma
   C.   Colon carcinoma
   D.   Renal cell carcinoma
   E.   Prostate carcinoma

722. In relation to what vessel are the cords of the brachial plexus named?
   A.   Brachiocephalic artery
   B.   Axillary artery
   C.   Subcalvian artery
   D.   Brachial artery
   E.   Internal carotid artery

723. Which type of spondylolisthesis is most common in gymnasts and football players?
   A.   Traumatic
   B.   Degenerative
   C.   Isthmic
   D.   Pathological
   E.   Dysplastic

Match the following visual disturbances with the choices that follow:
   A.   Homonymous hemianopia
   B.   Upper homonymous quadrantanopia
   C.   Bilateral central scotomas
   D.   Monocular loss of vision with contralateral upper outer quadrantanopia
   E.   Lower homonymous quadrantanopia

724. Lesion of the optic nerve just distal to the chiasm

725. Occipital lobe infarction

726. PICA interruption

727. Cushing's disease

728.   Temporal lobe lesion

729.   Parietal lobe lesion

Match the following anatomical structures with their related condition:
    A.   Struthers ligament
    B.   Arcade of Struthers
    C.   Arcade of Frohse
    D.   Guyon's canal

730.   Ulnar nerve entrapment

731.   Extensor carpi ulnaris palsy

732.   Brachial artery passes under this structure

733.   Which of the following is the LEAST likely presenting sign in a patient with rhinorrhea and this metrizamide CT scan finding?

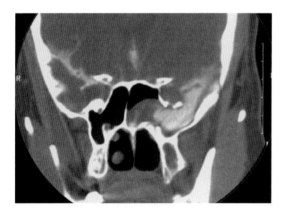

    A.   Reservoir sign
    B.   Early morning headache
    C.   Meningitis
    D.   Visual deficits
    E.   Sinus congestion

734.   Of the following signs and symptoms, which is the most common in the presentation of an osteoid osteoma of the spine?
    A.   Radicular pain
    B.   Scoliosis
    C.   Weakness
    D.   Atrophy
    E.   None of the above

735. Of the following signs and symptoms, which is the most common in the presentation of an osteoblastoma?
   A. Radicular pain
   B. Scoliosis
   C. Weakness
   D. Atrophy
   E. Cardiac ischemia

736. What mechanisms lead to neurological deficits in patients with vertebral hemangiomas?
   1. Epidural growth of the tumor
   2. Expansion of bone with widening of the pedicle and lamina
   3. Compression fracture of the involved vertebrae
   4. Spinal cord ischemia due to steal phenomenon
   A. 1, 2, and 3
   B. 1 and 3
   C. 2 and 4
   D. 1, 2, 3, and 4
   E. 2 and 3

737. DeQuervain's syndrome is characterized by all of the following EXCEPT:
   A. It is caused by frequent repetitive motion at the wrist.
   B. Pain and tenderness occurs in the wrist near the thumb.
   C. The Finkelstein test is positive.
   D. Nerve conduction velocities are decreased.
   E. There is difficulty with gripping.

Match the anatomical structure with its location:
   A. Fourth ventricle roof
   B. Fourth ventricle floor
   C. Both of the above
   D. None of the above

738. Inferior medullary velum

739. Facial colliculus

740. Hypoglossal trigone

741. Rhomboid fossa

742. What is the best therapeutic option in this 1-year-old with the lesion appearing on this MRI?

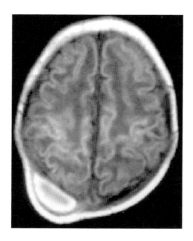

   A.   Surgical evacuation
   B.   Systemic antibiotics
   C.   Head wrapping
   D.   Radiation therapy
   E.   VP shunt

743. The dorsal horns of the spinal cord are derived from which of the following?
   A.   Basal plate
   B.   Notochord
   C.   Neural crest cells
   D.   Somites
   E.   Endoderm

Match the breathing pattern with the location of the lesion:
   A.   Cheyne–Stokes respiration
   B.   Apneustic respiration
   C.   Ataxic respiration
   D.   Central neurogenic hyperventilation

744. Medulla

745. Midbrain

746. Pons

747. Diencephalon

Match the cerebellar elements with their descriptions:
   A. Middle cerebellar peduncle
   B. Inferior cerebellar peduncle
   C. Nodulus
   D. Flocculus
   E. None of the above

748. Devoid of pontine inputs

749. Contains only afferent fibers

750. All the following are associated with this angiogram finding EXCEPT:

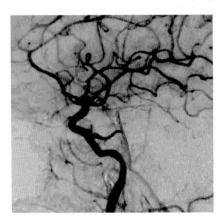

   A. It connects the basilar artery between the superior cerebellar and the anterior inferior cerebellar arteries by passing through the petrous bone.
   B. It connects the basilar artery by passing through the internal auditory meatus.
   C. It is present in 0.1% of the population.
   D. There is increased frequency of arteriovenous malformations.
   E. It is the second most common persistent fetal circulation.

Match the following risk rates with needlestick injury infections:
   A. 75%
   B. 50%
   C. 25%
   D. 2%
   E. 0.3%

751. The risk of acquiring HIV from a hollow needlestick injury from an affected individual

752. The risk of acquiring hepatitis C from a hollow needlestick injury from an affected individual

753. The risk of acquiring hepatitis B from a hollow needlestick injury from an affected individual with an extremely low viral load

754. This scan of a 35-year-old woman on hormonal contraceptives is most consistent with the diagnosis of

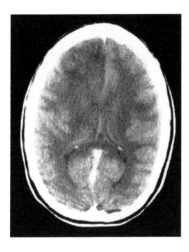

    A. tentorial subdural hemorrhage.
    B. subarachnoid hemorrhage.
    C. normal CT scan.
    D. dural sinus thrombosis.
    E. arteriovenous fistula.

755. All of the following are features of malignant hyperthermia EXCEPT:
    A. There is an autosomal recessive inheritance pattern.
    B. In 20% of cases there is no hyperthermia accompanying the muscle rigidity.
    C. It may be associated with autonomic instability.
    D. It may be caused by muscle relaxants.
    E. A mutation in the ryanodine receptor is related to malignant hyperthermia (MH).

756.   Which of the following is the lesion on this MRI scan associated with?

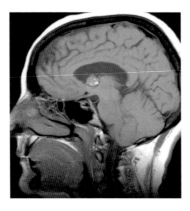

A.   Cerebral aneurysm
B.   Arteriovenous malformation
C.   Endocrinopathy
D.   Venous angioma
E.   Progressive supranuclear palsy

757.   Which of the following changes are represented at the end plates of L4–L5 levels on this T2-weighted MRI scan?

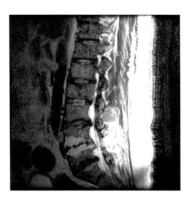

A.   Type 1 Modic changes
B.   Type 2 Modic changes
C.   Yellow marrow replacement
D.   Hypovascularization of the end plates
E.   None of the above

758. All of the following neurological deficits may be present with the lesion seen on this MRI scan EXCEPT:

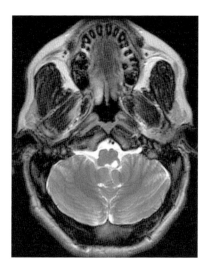

A. Ataxia
B. Ipsilateral hearing deficits
C. Contralateral temperature sensation loss
D. Lateral rectus palsy
E. Balance problems

759. Which anesthetic agent is least likely to cause further decrease in blood pressure in the face of hypovolemic shock?
A. Ketamine
B. Thiopental
C. Halothane
D. Enflurane
E. Isoflurane

760. Which of the following statements is not associated with the images shown here?

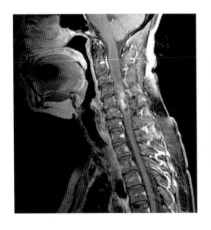 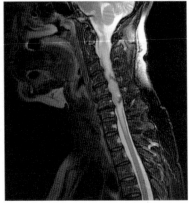

- **A.** Froin's syndrome
- **B.** Positive Queckenstedt's sign
- **C.** Male predominance with peak age in mid-40s
- **D.** Cellular type
- **E.** Neoplastic disease

761.   Which of the following is associated with this set of MRI scans in a patient with a functional ventriculoperitoneal shunt placed in the right ventricle?

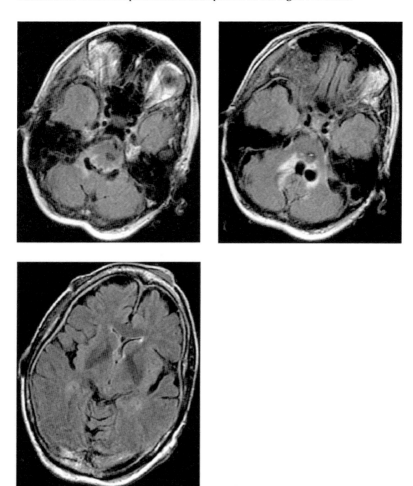

A.   Syringobulbia
B.   Elevated serum angiotensin-converting enzyme
C.   Aqueductal stenosis
D.   Hallervorden–Spatz disease
E.   Subdural hematoma

Match the following choices with their appropriate functions:
    A.   Proximal renal tubular function
    B.   Distal renal tubular function
    C.   Kidney glomerular function
    D.   None of the above

762.   Secretion of H^+ and reabsorption of Cl.

763.   Secretion of organic acids and reabsorption of amino acids

764.   Secretion of K^+ and reabsorption of Na^+

765.   Function is maximal in young adulthood and decreases thereafter.

766.   Which of the following prognostic factors is true in the case of a 16-year-old boy with failure to thrive and the following findings on MRI scan?

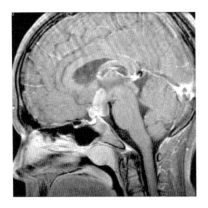 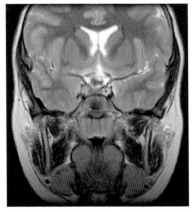

    A.   The most significant factor associated with recurrence is extent of resection.
    B.   A factor associated with recurrence is histology.
    C.   MIB-1 LI >7% is associated with a low likelihood of recurrence.
    D.   Malignant transformation to carcinoma frequently occurs.
    E.   Recurrence is dependent on the presence of intracytoplasmic inclusions.

767. This tumor shows on histopathology uniform round cells with perinuclear halos. Its immunohistochemistry is positive for synaptophysin. What is the most likely diagnosis?

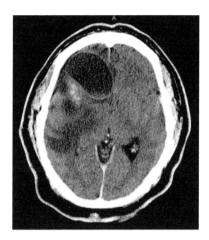

    A. Central neurocytoma
    B. Oligodendroglioma
    C. Ependymoma
    D. Endodermal sinus tumor
    E. Yolk sac tumor

768. The inferior frontal gyrus is bordered by which structure caudally?
    A. Operculum
    B. Sylvian fissure
    C. Precentral sulcus
    D. Rolandic fissure
    E. None of the above

769. The actions of nitroglycerine are mediated by the following mechanisms EXCEPT:
    A. Nitroglycerine binds the surface of endothelial cells.
    B. Nitroglycerine undergoes two chemical reductions to form nitric oxide.
    C. Nitric oxide promotes the formation of cyclic guanosine triphosphate.
    D. Nitric oxide moves out of the endothelial cell into adjacent smooth muscle cell.
    E. Nitric oxide increases cAMP in smooth muscle cells.

Match the closest relative risk of stroke with the appropriate patient presentation:
- **A.** 1% per year
- **B.** 2% per year
- **C.** 4% per year
- **D.** 13% per year
- **E.** 26% per year

770. Symptomatic 70–90% stenosis of the carotid on angiogram

771. Asymptomatic 70–90% stenosis of the carotid on angiogram

772. Postcarotid endarterectomy in a preoperative symptomatic 70–90% stenosis of the carotid on angiogram

773. Which of the following causes hypokalemia?
- **A.** Amphotericin
- **B.** Angiotensin-converting enzyme inhibitors
- **C.** Aspirin
- **D.** Cyclosporin
- **E.** Heparin

774. What is the most likely age of the hemorrhage shown here?

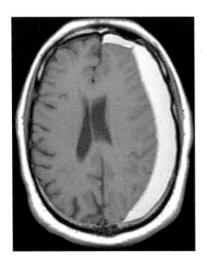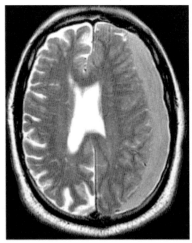

- **A.** 2 hours
- **B.** 2 days
- **C.** 12 days
- **D.** 22 days
- **E.** 32 days

Match the following substances with the choices:
A. Ethanol
B. Acetone
C. Methanol
D. Ethylene glycol (antifreeze)
E. Acethaldehyde

775. Lowest molecular weight

776. Most lethal

777. A patient with von Willebrand's disease sustained a motorcycle crash and is losing blood from an open fracture. The blood product best suited for management is
A. whole blood.
B. fibrinogen.
C. platelets.
D. packed red blood cells.
E. cryoprecipitate.

778. Which of the following is least likely to be associated with the finding on this MRI scan?

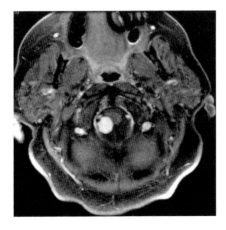

A. Ipsilateral Horner's syndrome
B. Downbeat nystagmus
C. Loss of abdominal cutaneous reflex
D. Neurogenic bladder
E. Extremity weakness

779. Typical presentation of patients with conus medullares lesions includes all of the following EXCEPT:
A. Saddle bilateral sensory deficit
B. Symmetric motor loss
C. Loss of ankle jerk
D. Autonomic symptoms that occur late
E. Urinary retention and atonic anal sphincter that cause overflow urinary incontinence and fecal incontinence

780. Typical presentation of patients with cauda equina lesions includes all of the following EXCEPT:
A. Sensory dissociation
B. Asymmetric motor loss
C. Late autonomic symptoms
D. Absence of ankle jerk and knee jerk
E. Numbness that tends to be more localized to saddle area

781. Which of the following structures is the second branch of the proximal aorta as it exits the left ventricle?
A. Brachiocephalic artery
B. Right subclavian artery
C. Left subclavian artery
D. Right carotid artery
E. Left carotid artery

782. Bilateral internuclear ophthalmoplegia results in which abnormality on physical exam?
A. Convergence deficit
B. Adduction deficit
C. Horizontal gaze palsy
D. Vertical gaze palsy
E. Parinaud's syndrome

Match the appropriate neurotransmitter with the area of the brain:
A. Acetylcholine
B. Noradrenaline
C. Dopamine
D. GABA
E. Glutamate

783. Inferior cervical ganglion

784. Locus ceruleus

785. Periaqueductal gray

786. In which disorder of speech are both repetition and comprehension affected?
   1. Transcortical sensory aphasia
   2. Wernicke's aphasia
   3. Conductive aphasia
   4. Global aphasia
A. 1, 2, and 3 are true.
B. 1 and 3 are true.
C. 2 and 4 are true.
D. Only 4 is true.
E. All of the above are true.

787. Watershed infarcts are seen in all of the following EXCEPT:
A. Regional hypotension
B. CBF below critical level
C. Atrial fibrillation
D. Cardiac arrest
E. Anaphylaxis

788. Which of the following arteries arises directly from the intracavernous carotid?
A. Bernasconi's artery
B. Persistent stapedial artery
C. Heubner's artery
D. McConnell's artery
E. Vidian artery

789. All the following statements are true regarding the findings of this scan EXCEPT:

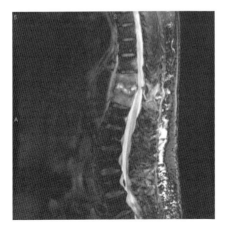

A. Thirty to fifty percent of patients are febrile.
B. Spontaneous fusion of vertebral bodies may occur.
C. *Haemophilus influenzae* may be a causative organism in juvenile cases.
D. Radionuclide scans have a relatively low sensitivity.
E. There is increased incidence with intravenous drug abuse.

790. What is the significance of an elevated N-acetylaspartate peak on an MR spectroscopy scan?
   A. Increased neuronal density
   B. Increased metabolism
   C. Increased excitatory neurotransmission
   D. Necrosis
   E. None of the above

Questions 791 and 792 are based on this radiograph:

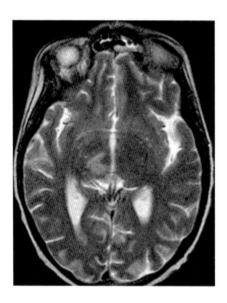

791. Choose the best answer based on the following MRI finding in a 20-year-old woman with Hodgkin's lymphoma and an opportunistic infection. Which of the following is the most likely infection?
   A. *Mucor*
   B. *Aspergillus*
   C. *Coccidioides*
   D. *E. histolytica*
   E. Virus

792. Characteristic features of the organism referred to in the preceding question include all of the following EXCEPT:
   A. Perivascular invasion
   B. Hemorrhagic infarcts
   C. Paranasal sinus mycetoma
   D. Caseating granulomas
   E. Increased prevalence with the use of chemotherapy and corticosteroids

793. What is the best treatment option in a 63-year-old woman with mental status changes and the following imaging study?

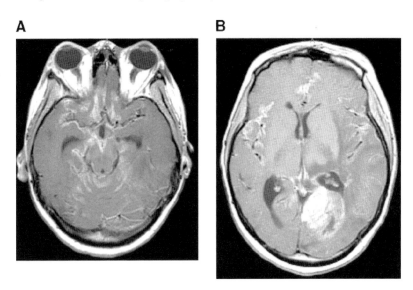

A   **B**

A.   Intravenous antibiotics
B.   Surgical resection
C.   Systemic chemotherapy and whole-brain radiation
D.   Ommaya reservoir placement and intrathecal chemotherapy
E.   Ventriculoperitoneal shunt

794. Which of the following muscles is innervated by the glossopharyngeal nerve?
A.   Stapedius
B.   Tensor veli palatini
C.   Stylopharyngeus
D.   Posterior belly of digastric
E.   None of the above

Match the following choices with the appropriate measurements on the lung volume spirogram:

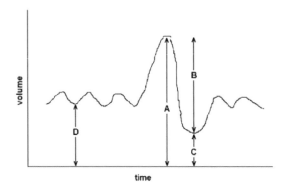

795.   Equals 2.4 L at rest and 2.4 L during exercise

796.   Represents vital capacity minus expiratory reserve volume

797.   Measured at ~4.4 to 5 L in healthy adults

798.   Calculated after having the patient inspire a mixture containing 10% helium from a spirometer at 21°C

Questions 799 and 800 are based on this MR spectroscopy study:

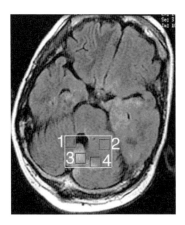
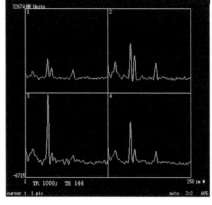

799. Point 1 being closest to normal and point 3 showing the most abnormality, which of the following statements with regard to spectroscopy is correct regarding point 3?

  A. Elevated N-acetylaspartate (NAA) peak and normal choline (Chol) and creatine (Cr) peaks

  B. Elevated Cr peak and decreased Chol and NAA peaks

  C. Increased Chol:Cr ratio and decreased NAA peak

  D. Increased Cr:Chol ratio and decreased NAA peak

  E. All of the above

800. What do the preceding MR spectroscopy findings most likely represent?

  A. Increased astrocytic density at point 3 as compared with point 1

  B. Presence of tumor cells at point 3

  C. Presence of necrosis at point 3

  D. Increased metabolism at point 3

  E. All of the above

801. Which of the following is represented by X in this formula?

  $X = $ (Cardiac output) (Arterial O_2 content – venous O_2 content)

  A. Oxygen delivery

  B. Oxygen uptake

  C. Oxygen extraction ratio

  D. Oxygen content

  E. None of the above

802. Which of the following formulas describes shunt fraction?

  Note:

  Pulmonary capillary O_2 content = $Cc\,O_2$

  Venous O_2 content = $Cv\,O_2$

  Arterial O_2 content = $Ca\,O_2$

  A. $Cc\,O_2 - Ca\,O_2 \,/\, Cv\,O_2 - Ca\,O_2$

  B. $(Cc\,O_2 - Cv\,O_2)/(Cc\,O_2 - Ca\,O_2)$

  C. $Cc\,O_2 - Ca\,O_2/Cc\,O_2 - Cv\,O_2$

  D. $(Cc\,O_2 - Ca\,O_2)/(Cc\,O_2 - Cv\,O_2)$

  E. $(Cc\,O_2 - Ca\,O_2)/(Cv\,O_2 - Ca\,O_2)$

803.   Which of the following is the formula for flow (Q) of nonpulsatile fluids?
Note:

        P = pressure
        R = radius
        L = length
        V = viscosity

A. $Q = P\pi r^4/8VL$
B. $Q = 8PL/V\pi r^4$
C. $Q = V\pi r^4/8PL$
D. $Q = 8V\pi r^4/PL$
E.   None of the above

804.   A prisoner with suicidal tendencies is brought to the emergency room after stabbing himself in the eye with a pencil. The patient is started on broad-spectrum antibiotics, antiseizure medication, and taken immediately for open surgical debridement. The CT scan shown here is taken. The foreign object should be removed

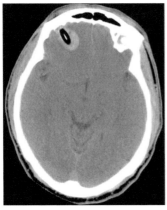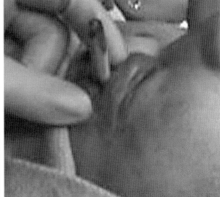

A.   immediately in the ER.
B.   before a CT scan.
C.   in the operating room.
D.   before antibiotics are given.
E.   after the patient has been stabilized.

805.   A 48-year-old woman presents with progressive myelopathy and difficulty walking for several months. Her MRI and CT scans are shown here. What would be the best management of the offending lesion?

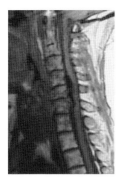 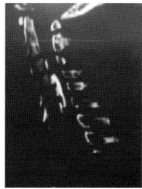

A.   Single-level anterior cervical diskectomy and fusion (ACDF)
B.   Two-level ACDF
C.   Posterior decompression
D.   Cervical corpectomy and fusion
E.   Three-level ACDF

Answers

1.D. All three are mechanisms of anti-acetylcholine receptor antibodies.

2.B. The medial lemniscus (ML) is widely separated from the anterolateral system (ALS) in the medulla. In fact, ML and ALS fibers receive different blood supplies in the medulla. In the midbrain and pons, the ML and ALS are in close proximity and receive similar blood supplies.

3.D. The CT scan represents sclerosis of the sacroiliac (SI) joint, which may be seen in ankylosing spondylosis. This is representative of the diagnosis of sacroiliitis. Clinically the patient usually presents with SI joint pain and on exam has tenderness along the SI joint with compression as well as a positive thigh thrust and thigh compression exam and a positive flexion, abduction, and external rotation (FABER) test. Pain upon internal rotation of the hip is characteristic of hip joint dysfunction or disease.

4.A. McRae's line is from the basion to the opisthion.

5.C. It is helpful to remember that this pattern of somatotopy can be appreciated in the descending motor pathways: those that are concerned with flexor musculature (corticospinal tract and rubrospinal tract) lie dorsal to those tracts concerned with extensor musculature.

6.D. Although skin surface fiducial registration is commonly used in brain neuronavigation, it is not very effective in the spine due to the parallax that is seen from registering on the skin and attempting to navigate at the level of the bone, which tends to be significantly deeper than the level of the skin. The other techniques described for localization are effective in identifying the level of interest in that the thoracic spine adequately.

7.A. Rhinocerebral mucormycosis on pathology reveals pleomorphic short and wide nonseptate hyphae. It can be treated with Cancidas, voriconazole, and AmBisome. It may cause hemorrhagic necrosis and ischemic strokes.

8.B. Somatic motor efferents to the sphincter are located in the ventral lateral area of Onuf's nucleus. Sacral parasympathetics to the bladder are located in intermediolateral cell columns of the sacral cord. Barrington's nucleus is also known as the pontine micturition center and is responsible for initiating the process of micturition.

9.C. Cerebral ischemia begins when CPP falls below 50 mm Hg.

10.B. The clinoidal triangle is defined by the medial border of the optic nerve medially and the oculomotor nerve laterally.

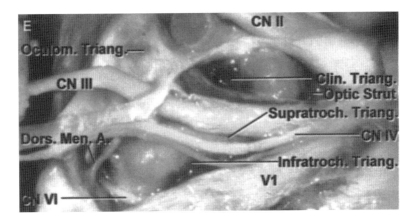

11.E. Dysphagia in myasthenia gravis is fatigable, and the patient often relates a history of little difficulty with breakfast, moderate difficulty with lunch, and inability to eat in the evening.

12.E. Skin changes precede muscle abnormalities in dermatomyositis (DM). Poly-myositis (PM) is diagnosed by fibrillation potentials on electromyography (EMG) and elevated creatine phosphokinase (CPK) levels (higher than those for DM). In polymyositis, there is widespread single-fiber necrosis, and T cells with macrophages may be found in the muscle fibers. PM is the most frequent inflammatory myopathy.

13.E. *Protein 14-3-3* is elevated in the cerebrospinal fluid (CSF) with destructive diseases of the central nervous system (CNS). This protein is sensitive for Creutzfeldt-Jakob disease, but not specific.

14.B. The posterior cord gives rise to the axillary nerve and the radial nerve as its terminal branches.

15.C. The pterion is located about two fingerbreadths above the zygomatic arch, and a thumb's breadth behind the frontal process of the zygomatic bone; however, the zygomatic bone does not form the pterion.

16.D. SHH has been found to have the critical roles in development of the limb and midline structures in the brain and spinal cord. Mutations in the human SHH gene cause holoprosencephaly type 3 as a result of the loss of the ventral mid-line. SHH is secreted at the zone of polarizing activity located on the posterior side of a limb bud in an embryo. The SHH transcription pathway has also been linked to the formation of embryonic cerebellar tumors such as medulloblasto-ma. SHH has been shown to act as an axonal guidance cue: SHH attracts retinal ganglion cell axons at low concentrations and repels them at higher concentra-tions. SHH plays a critical role in the induction of the floor plate and diverse ventral cell types within the neural tube.

17.D. After basilar skull fractures, the most common pathogen is *Streptococcus pneu-moniae*, and the infection usually occurs within the first few days.

18.C. The zona incerta is a zone of gray matter between the thalamic and lenticu-lar fasciculi. It is composed of cells that are continuous laterally with the tha-lamic reticular nucleus. Unlike the thalamic reticular nucleus, the neurons of this zone display immunoreactivity for the calcium binding protein calbindin D-28k. It receives corticofugal fibers from the precentral cortex.

19.A. While lower cranial nerve dysfunction may be a relative contraindication for vagal nerve stimulation, upper cranial nerve deficits do not represent such a contraindication.

20.D.

21.B.

22.E. Weber's syndrome involves the base of the midbrain. It is characterized by CN III palsy with crossed hemiplegia. All other syndromes mentioned may have ataxia as part of the clinical findings.

23.E.

24.C. Lesions of the dorsomedial nucleus of the thalamus, hippocampus, or temporal cortex cause memory impairment.

25.B. The X-ray shows a cervical rib, usually associated with ulnar nerve weakness and paresthesia, Raynaud's syndrome, and traction meningocele.

26.E. Bannayan–Riley–Ruvalcaba's syndrome (BRRS) is a rare overgrowth disorder with occurrence of multiple subcutaneous lipomas, macrocephaly, and hemangiomas. The disease is inherited in an autosomal dominant fashion, but sporadic cases have been seen. The syndrome belongs to a family of hamartomatous polyposis syndromes, which includes Peutz–Jeghers's syndrome, juvenile polyposis, and Cowden disease. Mutation of the PTEN gene is associated with this syndrome, Cowden disease, Proteus syndrome, and Proteus-like syndrome. These four syndromes are referred to as PTEN hamartoma-tumor syndromes. Intracranial arteriovenous malformations represent a rare feature of BRRS. Capillary malformation or "port-wine stain," is a cutaneous vascular anomaly that initially appears as a red macular stain that darkens over time. It also occurs in several combined vascular anomalies that exhibit hypertrophy, such as Sturge–Weber's syndrome and Klippel–Trénaunay's syndrome.

27.B. The external capsule is located between the claustrum and the putamen. The extreme capsule is located between the claustrum and the insular cortex.

28.B. Serotonin pathways inhibit copulation, explaining the side effect of decreased libido with selective serotonin reuptake inhibitors (SSRIs) used to treat depression. Administration of L-dopa increases libido. Noradrenergic receptors in the brain exert an inhibitory effect on penile erection.

29.E. The peak reduction in intracranial pressure (ICP) occurs in about 15 minutes after administration of mannitol. The duration of action of mannitol is about 4 hours due to the rapid renal elimination of the drug. When mannitol is used with furosemide, the combined effect on ICP reduction is greater than if either were used alone.

30.C. The paramedial triangle (also known as the supratrochlear triangle) is defined medially by the medial border of the oculomotor nerve and laterally by the lateral border of the trochlear nerve.

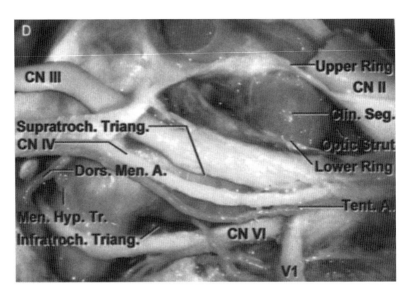

31.D. The Tensilon test is sensitive in diagnosing a defect in neuromuscular transmission but is not specific for myasthenia gravis (MG). The Tensilon test is especially useful in ocular MG, when other diagnostic tests may be negative. Depending on the mechanism of acetylcholine receptor (AchR) antibodies, there may be insufficient numbers of AchRs available so that a negative Tensilon test does not negate the diagnosis of MG. There is no correlation between the results of the Tensilon test and the subsequent response to pyridostigmine.

32.D. The posterior interosseous nerve (C7, C8) is a branch of the radial nerve. The posterior interosseous nerve innervates the extensor digitorum, extensor digiti minimi, and extensor carpi ulnaris. The extensor carpi ulnaris extends the hand at the wrist joint. This muscle is spared in posterior interosseous syndrome.

33.B. The magnetic resonance angiography scan (MRA) represents the findings of a left anterior frontal arteriovenous malformation (AVM) of which the nidus measures between 3 and 6 cm, which adds two points in the Spetzler–Martin grading system. It is located in noneloquent brain and has superficial drainage; therefore it is a grade 2 Spetzler–Martin AVM.

34.B. Interruption of the inferior geniculocalcarine fibers in the temporal lobe produces a "pie in the sky" deficit (contralateral superior quadrantanopia).

35.D. Ocular myoclonus is a pendular vertical oscillation of the eyes, usually of large amplitude and often occurring with movements of the palate. It can develop months to years after bilateral destructive lesions of the central tegmental tract and is often accompanied by bilateral horizontal gaze palsies and is associated with hypertrophy of the inferior olivary nucleus.

36.A. Early hypoxemia characterizes ARDS.

37.C. Maximum collagen deposition occurs at 42 days (about 6 weeks). Tensile strength keeps on increasing until 2 years.

38.B. Rosenthal fibers are by no means a requisite feature of pilocytic astrocytoma. Rosenthal fibers are composed of *alpha B* cystallin and are surrounded by intermediate filaments.

39.E. Barbiturates are also thought to stabilize lysosomes, suppress the formation of edema, and reduce intracellular accumulation of calcium. The inverse steal phenomenon involves barbiturate-induced vasoconstriction resulting in shunting of blood from normal brain to relatively ischemic areas.

40.C. Parkinson's triangle is also known as the infratrochlear triangle.

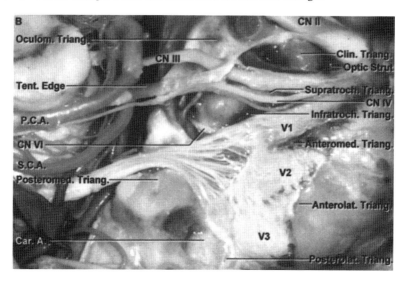

41.C. The majority of acetylcholine receptor (AchR) antibodies are immunoglobulin G (IgG). Cyclosporine should be used once first-line treatments have failed. Pathological abnormalities of the thymus occur in up to 80% of patients. Weakness confined to the ocular muscles for over 3 years suggests good prognosis.

42.D.

43.E. Tolosa–Hunt syndrome is characterized by ocular and retro-orbital pain, ocular motor paralysis (with papillary sparing), and possibly sensory loss over the forehead with granulomatous inflammation of the superior orbital fissure or the lateral wall of the cavernous sinus. The other conditions described lack an inflammatory response.

44.B. The most accurate description of Wernicke's area is that it includes the supramarginal (39), angular (40), and posterior one-third of the superior temporal gyri.

45.A. Bursts of back-to-back saccades seen in opsoclonus and ocular flutter may be attributable to a disorder of pause cell modulation of burst cell function.

46.C.

47.A.   Scan 1 shows a glomus tympanicum tumor, which may be associated with
48.B.   catecholamine release causing hypertension, or serotonin and kallikrein
49.A.   release causing bronchoconstriction, abdominal pain, and explosive di-
50.A.   arrhea. Glomus tympanicum tumors may also release histamine and
51.D.   bradykinins during surgery causing hypotension and bronchoconstriction. Scan 2 shows a meningioma of the cerebellopontine angle (CPA), which usually presents initially with facial nerve involvement. Acoustic schwannomas present initially with hearing loss and tinnitus.

52.A. Disseminated intravascular coagulation (DIC) is most frequently associated with obstetric catastrophes, metastatic malignancy, massive trauma, and bacterial sepsis. The neurosurgeon should be aware that DIC can occur when there is major cerebral tissue injury. The decrease in fibrinogen most closely correlates with increased bleeding. Treatment is by removing the causative agent, heparin, cryoprecipitate, platelets, and whole blood.

53.C. The mastoid air cells and the posterior middle fossa are innervated by V_3. The supratentorial compartment is innervated by V_1 and V_2. The infratentorial compartment is innervated by IX, X, and C1–C3 posterior roots.

54.D. The band of Gennari divides the fourth layer of cortex into two granular layers with a thick myelin layer. The band is located only in area 17 (primary visual cortex, also known as V_1). When Gennari described this in 1782, he had no idea that this or any other region of the visual cortex might be concerned with vision.

55.E. The neural integrator for horizontal eye movements is located in the nucleus prepositus hypoglossi (NPH) at the pontomedullary junction.

56.C. Climbing fiber input is most active at times when the subject is performing new complex movements. The climbing fiber input can modify the synapse between the parallel fiber (from the granule cell) and the Purkinje cell.

57.D. The combination of high trophic hormone and low target hormone indicates target gland failure.

58.D. The opponens pollicis inserts on the first metacarpal bone.

59.C. The MRI with contrast demonstrates a left cerebellopontine angle lesion most consistent with a vestibular schwannoma. Most patients have involvement of the eighth cranial nerve initially. They may also more commonly present with decreased facial sensation or numbness with involvement of the trigeminal nerve; however, facial nerve involvement with a tumor of the size shown is relatively uncommon.

60.B.
61.C.
62.A.
63.E.
64.D.

65.C. The medial longitudinal fasciculus (MLF) is responsible for the binocular co-ordination of all categories of horizontal, vertical, and oblique eye movements with the exception of vergence movements. Upbeating nystagmus on upgaze is a feature of MLF lesions.

66.C. Both Apert's and Crouzon's syndromes are autosomal dominant (both may also be sporadic). Both are associated with bilateral coronal synostosis. Patients with Apert's syndrome manifest more severe mental retardation than patients with Crouzon's syndrome.

67.E. In addition to stimulating the synthesis and secretion of thyroid stimulating hormone (TSH), thyrotropin-releasing hormone (TRH) is a potent secretagogue for prolactin, and to a lesser extent adrenocorticotropic hormone (ACTH), and growth hormone (GH).

68.C. The metacarpophalangeal joint of the ring finger is flexed by the lumbrical, pal-mar, and dorsal interosseous muscles, which are innervated by the ulnar nerve. The joint is extended by the extensor digitorum, which is innervated by the ra-dial nerve. The median nerve is mainly involved with flexion of the ring finger.

69.E. Profile expression:
Survivin—83%
MMP-9—69%
EGFR—63%
MDM2—31%
Fas (APO-1/CD95)—100%

70.D.

71.E. Serum concentration of prolactin (PRL) is increased after tonicoclonic seizure activity but is not affected by nonepileptic seizures.

72.D. The subfornical organ is located on the inferior surface of the fornix at the level of the foramen of Monro.

73.A. The sinuvertebral nerve arises just distal to the dorsal root ganglion. The posterior disk receives its innervation from the sinuvertebral nerves. The anterior disk receives its innervation from the gray rami communicans.

74.B. Repetition is impaired in conduction aphasia.

75.B. The usual diameter of the internal cerebral artery at the clinoid area is about 8 mm. This aneurysm is slightly smaller than the artery's diameter.

76.C. The Torg-Pavlov ratio is a measure of cervical spinal stenosis and is the ratio of spinal canal to vertebral body. A normal cervical spinal canal will have a ratio of about 1.0. A stenotic cervical canal has a ratio of <0.8.

77.B. Primary glioblastoma has an incidence that is about 10 times higher than secondary glioblastoma. The mean age at presentation in secondary glioblastoma is much younger (45 years) than in primary glioblastoma (62 years). Primary glioblastoma is more common in males when compared to secondary glioblastoma. The median survival at presentation is longer in secondary glioblastoma as compared to primary glioblastoma. Loss of heterozygosity on 10p or 10q is one of the most common genetic mutations in primary glioblastoma.

78.C. The medial brachial cutaneous nerve (from the medial cord) contains sensory fibers that have cell bodies in the dorsal root ganglia. It also contains sympathetic postganglionic fibers that have cell bodies in the sympathetic chain ganglia.

79.B. The perforant path is the main excitatory pathway to the hippocampus. When perforant path fibers are stimulated, histological changes develop in the pyramidal nerve cells of CA1 and CA3.

80.D.

81.B. Up to 80% of the population will experience a tension headache in their lifetime. Amitriptyline is the most effective medication used to prevent tension headaches.

82.C. The ambient cistern contains the trochlear nerve.

83.B. The anterior and medial scalene muscles insert onto the first rib, and the subclavian artery, subclavian vein, and brachial plexus pass between them.

84.A. Pure word blindness is characterized by alexia without agraphia. The patient is unable to read but is able to understand speech, write, and speak. It is caused by a lesion of the left geniculocalcarine tract and the corpus callosum.

85.C. Preventing seepage of blood into the ventricular system during a hemispherectomy is accomplished by obstructing the foramen of Monro and maintaining the integrity of the septum pellucidum.

86.A. Experiments in functional physiology defined a limited role of the horizontal fibers and reinforced the anatomical principles of vertical columnar organization in the cortex. This functional columnar organization of cortical architecture is the key principle in multiple subpial transection.

87.D. Sexual precocity is often the presenting symptom of hypothalamic hamartomas. Hamartomas may also cause gelastic (laughing) seizures.

88.D. Pleomorphic xanthoastrocytoma (PXA) is an astrocytic neoplasm with a relatively favorable prognosis.

89.B. Excitatory input from CA3 to CA1 pyramidal cells is carried by Schaffer collaterals. These collaterals spare the CA2 region.

90.B. The MRI scan of the lumbar spine demonstrates a far lateral foraminal disk herniation at L4–L5 on the left side. Most likely, the L4 nerve root will be involved and the patient will present with weakness of the tibialis anterior and decreased sensation along an L4 distribution in the left lower extremity.

91.B. Although a midline laminotomy or laminectomy may be employed for decompression and removal of the disk it is often more effective to approach the disk via a direct approach that is paramedian with a partial facetectomy in order to remove the foraminal and extraforaminal portions.

92.D. The gracile and cuneate fasciculi are supplied by the posterior spinal arteries. The paired posterior spinal arteries (arising from either the posterior inferior cerebellar artery (PICA) or vertebral artery) supply the posterior one-third of the spinal cord.

93.C. Adson's test is used in the examination of thoracic outlet syndrome. In this example the examiner is checking to see if the radial pulse is obliterated. Compression of nerves causes wasting of muscles supplied by the lower trunk of the brachial plexus.

94.E. The corticobulbar tract is located in the genu of the internal capsule.

95.D. The medial forebrain bundle traverses the entire lateral hypothalamic area and interconnects the septal area and nuclei, the hypothalamus, and the midbrain tegmentum. The medulla is connected with the hypothalamus via the dorsal longitudinal fasciculus, which projects to the parasympathetic nuclei of the brainstem.

96.D. It is postulated that the closure of the lambdoid sutures, common in Crouzon's syndrome, results in cerebellar tonsillar herniation.

97.A. The most severe forms of hypothalamic cachexia are seen in lesions of the lateral hypothalamus.

98.C. Lesions of the prefrontal cortex result in a failure to discriminate odors. The prefrontal cortex receives projections from the pyriform cortex. There is also a projection from the pyriform cortex to the dorsomedial thalamus to the prefrontal cortex.

99.A. The amino acids phenylalanine and tyrosine are precursors for catecholamines (dopamine, norepinephrine, epinephrine).

100.D. Renal cell carcinoma has a predilection to the ventricular system.

101.B. The majority of cases of glioblastomas are primary that develop without clinical or histological evidence of a less malignant precursor lesion. They occur primarily in the elderly and typically present genetically with loss of heterozygosity 10q, EGFR amplification, $p16^{INK4a}$ deletion, and PTEN mutations. Secondary glioblastomas occur through progression from low-grade diffuse astrocytoma or anaplastic astrocytoma and tend to present in younger patients. TP53 mutations are the most frequent in the pathways to these tumors being often present in precursor low-grade astrocytomas.

102.B.   The straight sinus is formed by the great cerebral vein (of Galen) and the inferior sagittal sinus.

103.D.   Oscillopsia is a condition where objects seem to wiggle; it sometimes accompanies downbeat nystagmus.

104.A.   Atropine blocks only muscarinic receptors, thus only preganglionic synapses are affected.

105.A.   Wernicke's encephalopathy is due to deficiency of thiamine (B_1).

106.D.   Gustatory fibers of the solitary nucleus terminate in the VPM. Fibers carrying thoracic information travel via solitary tract and terminate in the parabrachial nucleus and hypothalamus.

107.B.   In contrast to diffuse astrocytomas, anaplastic astrocytomas typically display mitotic activity.

108.D.   The typical site for a cavernous hemangioma of the orbit is in the intraconal space lateral to the optic nerve.

109.D.   HIV-infected individuals have an increased risk of cerebrovascular incidents associated with intravenous drug abuse, low CD4 cell count, and exposure to abacavir, but not with HAART. A CD4 cell count ≤ 200 cells/mL prior the start of HAART increased the risk of cerebrovascular events.

110.E.   Arteries from the ependymal surface feed the arteriovenous malformation (AVM).

111.A.   Under conditions of neuronal activation, dopamine beta-hydroxylase is the rate-limiting step. However, under basal conditions tyrosine hydroxylase is the rate-limiting step.

112.B.   The venous angle is a landmark of the foramen of Monro. It is formed by the union of the septal vein and the terminal (also called thalamostriate) vein.

113.E.   Ocular bobbing is a rapid downward movement of the eyes with a slow return to midposition and has many causes.

114.E.   This CT scan reveals dense sclerosis around a lytic lesion with a central calcified nodule in the lumbar neural arch consistent with osteoid osteoma.

115.C. The striae *medullares* (rhombencephali) arise from the arcuate nuclei of the medulla and are seen on the floor of the rhomboid fossa. These fibers divide the rhomboid fossa into a rostral pontine half and a caudal medullary half. The stria *medullaris* (thalami) contains septohabenular fibers. The stria terminalis is a semicircular fiber bundle extending from the amygdala to the hypothalamus and septal area.

116.C. No blood vessels penetrate the intervertebral disk. Delivery of nutrients is entirely dependent on diffusion.

117.D. The olivocochlear bundle arises from the region of the superior olivary nucleus and projects contralaterally back to the hair cells of the cochlea. Stimulation of this bundle results in inhibition or reduction of responses of auditory signals by auditory nerve fibers.

118.B. Pleomorphic adenomas of the lacrimal gland should be removed with a cuff of normal tissue to reduce the risk of tumor seeding and recurrence. An incisional biopsy should not be performed on this type of tumor.

119.C.

120.C.

121.C. Hydromyelia has ependymal lining. It can be associated with both hydrocephalus and Chiari but can also be postmeningitic and associated with tumors. It can be either communicating with the fourth ventricle or just isolated and noncommunicating. Syrinxes on the other hand lack any ependymal lining.

122.B. The superior cerebellar artery supplies the superior surface of the cerebellum and the cerebellar nuclei.

123.D. In the comatose patient, a lesion at the level of the vestibular nuclei results in extensor movements of the arms and weak flexor movements of the legs. Flaccidity of the lower and upper extremities occurs with lesions below the vestibular nuclei. Lesions above the red nucleus (*decorticate*) result in flexion of the upper and extension of the lower extremities. Lesions below the red nucleus (and above the vestibular nuclei) result in extensor posturing of all extremities (*decerebrate*).

124.E. Fibers of the chorda tympani reach the sphenopalatine ganglion to produce "crocodile tears," also known as Bogorad's syndrome.

125.A. With a cervical syrinx, one would expect attenuation or abolition of the cervical N13 evoked potential. N13 attenuation may be due to involvement of those laminae of the dorsal horn that receive input from large-diameter mechano-receptor fibers.

126.C. Wolff's law states that a bone develops the structure most suited to resist the forces acting upon it. Sherrington's law: every posterior spinal nerve supplies a special region of skin. Jackson's law: the nerve functions that are latest developed are the first to be lost. Delpech's principle: in spondylolisthesis, when slippage reaches around 30% the anterior inferior part grows at a faster rate than the overloaded posterior part of the vertebral body. Flourens' law deals with nystagmus, not spine biomechanics.

127.D. Chordomas tend to be in the midline, whereas chondrosarcomas are more frequently found off the midline (at the petrosphenoid synchondrosis). Chordomas express S-100 only variably. Normal neurological examinations are more common in patients with chordoma, whereas visual loss, facial numbness, and multiple cranial neuropathies are more common in patients with chondrosarcoma. These differences probably reflect the tendency of chordomas to originate from the clivus and chondrosarcomas from the temporal bone.

128.A. Thalamotomy is quite effective for medically refractory essential tremor. The Parkinson's patients who benefit most from thalamotomy are usually young, with tremor-predominant Parkinson's disease.

129.D. Due to considerable variation in the attachment of the dentate ligament, the best estimate of the equator is the midway point of the dorsal and ventral rootlets. The equator is a useful landmark for the posterior extent of a cordotomy incision and marks the point of the sacralmost fibers of the spinothalamic tract. The exiting ventral root is about 5 mm from the anterior spinal artery.

130.C. It usually takes 12 to 18 months for radiation changes to appear on MRI scans.

131.C. L-dopa is converted very quickly to dopamine by aromatic L-amino acid decarboxylase (AADC). Dopamine is converted to norepinephrine (NE) by dopamine beta hydroxylase, which is found in vesicles within the catecholaminergic neuron.

132.B.

133.A.   The length constant is the distance along a fiber where a change in the membrane potential produced by a given current decays to a value of approximately one-third of its original value. It is directly proportional to membrane resistance and inversely related to axial resistance (the resistance of the cytoplasm within the fiber).

134.D.   Raynaud's phenomenon is caused by mast cell dysfunction; sympathectomy has not proven helpful. Half of these patients have collagen vascular disease.

135.D.   Epidural hematomas are the most common intracranial hematoma in children. Although an arterial component is of major concern, diffuse oozing from the bone or from the highly vascularized periosteal surface of the dura is now considered to be a more common source of epidural hematomas in children.

136.E.   Spondylolysis is a bone defect in the posterior vertebral arch between the upper and lower articular processes, that is, the isthmus or pars interarticularis.

137.B.   Winged scapula is caused by paralysis of the serratus anterior muscle as a result of damage to the long thoracic nerve that arises from the roots of the brachial plexus (C5–C7).

138.A.   The typical thalamotomy target is the Vim (ventralis intermedius) nucleus. Often just inserting the electrode into Vim reduces the tremor (microthalamotomy effect), and indicates that the electrode is in a good position.

139.D.   All are derived from the telencephalon.

140.D.

141.E.   The MRI represents thoracic diskitis at a midthoracic level. Oftentimes this can be treated medically. Indications for surgery, however, do include failure of medical treatments, requirement for identification of offending agent via biopsy, mass effect caused by compression of the cord, or instability that is caused by an abscess or significant bony destruction. Sensory deficit alone is not a clear indication for surgical intervention.

142.B.

143.D.   The spiral ganglion consists of bipolar neurons of the cochlear division of the vestibulocochlear nerve.

144.E. The supplementary motor area (area 6) is unique because a lesion in that location is associated with no language output, usually with complete recovery in weeks to months. This is in contrast with the perisylvian language sites.

145.A. During middle fossa approaches, this anatomy can be appreciated. As the dura is elevated, branches of the middle meningeal artery are encountered, and the greater and lesser superficial petrosal nerves are identified immediately posterior to the foramen spinosum. With careful bone removal, the greater superficial petrosal nerve can be traced back to the geniculate ganglion.

146.E. The position of the posterior inferior tip of L5 above one of the quarters characterizes grade I, II, III, or IV spondylolisthesis, respectively (III–V being higher grades).

147.D. Golgi tendon organs detect tension in the muscle fiber. Afferent signals are carried by Ib fibers to interneurons that decrease the alpha motor neuron output.

148.D. The ventralis intermedius (Vim) is thought to be a relay nucleus for kinesthetic sensation. All observations indicate placement in the Vim. Contralateral paresthesias from stimulation of the Vim occur at higher thresholds than those obtained from the ventralis caudalis (VC) nucleus (posterior to the Vim).

149.C. Glomeruli of the olfactory nerve are composed of mitral and tufted cells. Axons of mitral and tufted cells go on to form the lateral olfactory tract.

150.A. The sylvian triangle is defined angiographically by (1) the most posterior branch of the middle cerebral artery as it exits the sylvian fissure, (2) branches of superior ramifications of the MCA, and (3) inferior loops of the MCA.

151.D. MAO_A and MAO_B are associated with the outer mitochondrial membrane.

152.A. The metencephalon is a secondary vesicle that becomes the pons, cerebellum, and upper part of the fourth ventricle. The myelencephalon becomes the medulla and the lower part of the fourth ventricle.

153.A. The tectorial membrane is a projection of the spiral limbus that overlies hair cells of the organ of Corti. The basilar membrane supports the organ of Corti and separates the cochlear duct from the scala tympani. The vestibular (Reissner's membrane) separates the scala vestibuli from the cochlear duct.

154.B. Solitary projections to the nucleus ambiguus are largely bilateral and are the intermediate neurons in the pathway for the gag reflex.

155.C.   The film shows a grade I spondylolisthesis at L4–L5. Although management of this problem is wide ranging, from the choices given the best management is a pedicle screw fusion at the concerning levels (L4–L5).

156.B.   The GABA-B receptor is activated by the GABA analogue baclofen, is not chloride dependent, and is bicuculline insensitive. GABA-C is found in the retina, hippocampus, and cerebellum, and is insensitive to baclofen and bicuculline.

157.C.   Structures that pass above the tendinous ring are the lacrimal nerve, frontal nerve, and CN IV (trochlear).

158.C.   The most common causative organism of brain abscesses in trauma is *Staphylococcus.*

159.B.   The most common causative organism of brain abscesses in adults due to chronic otitis is *Streptococcus.*

160.A.   The most common causative organisms of brain abscesses in neonates are *Citrobacter, Bacteroides, Proteus* and gram-negative bacilli.

161.A.   Tranylcypromine is an inhibitor of MAO_A. Deprenyl is a specific inhibitor of MAO_B.

162.B.   The floor plate contains the ventral white commissure.

163.E.   Sturge–Weber syndrome occurs sporadically without Mendelian inheritance and is of unknown etiology.

164.E.   There are nonchoroid plexus sites of cerebrospinal fluid (CSF) production. Likewise there are sites of absorption other than the arachnoid granulations (paranasal sinuses, cervical lymphatics, exiting nerve roots, and transependymal flow).

165.C.   In patients with known systemic cancer, 10–15% of single brain lesions are cerebral abscesses or primary brain tumors.

166.A.   Vigabatrin interferes with GABA breakdown, whereas tiagabine interferes with GABA reuptake.

167.B.

168.B. Lesions placed too laterally during thalamotomy risk injury to the internal capsule (posterior limb). Lesions placed too posterior may cause contralateral hemisensory deficits owing to injury of the ventralis caudalis (VC) nucleus.

169.B. Cyclosporine along with some of the newer immunosuppressive agents (FK-506 or tacrolimus) work at the level of the T cells by inhibiting expression of IL-2.

170.E. The perforating arteries from the Pcom are termed the *anterior thalamo-perforating* arteries. Those from the P1 are called the *posterior thalamo-perforating* arteries. Those from P2 are termed the *thalamo-geniculate* arteries.

171.D.

172.E. The basal plate gives rise to the hypoglossal nucleus, nucleus ambiguus, dorsal motor nucleus of the vagal nerve, and inferior salivatory nucleus.

173.B.

174.B. Kocher's point places the catheter in the frontal horn of the lateral ventricle. One can measure 1 cm anteriorly to the coronal suture or 3.5 cm in front of the bregma. This precaution is to avoid the motor strip. Keen's point would be used for placement of the catheter in the trigone and would require entrance through the posterior parietal region.

175.B. The MRI demonstrates absent flow voids in the left vertebral artery, a finding seen in Wallenberg syndrome.

176.C. Clonazepam acts by increasing GABA-A opening frequency and does not have any hepatic enzyme–inducing properties.

177.A.

178.E. Freezing episodes and postural instability do not appear to be improved with pallidotomy.

179.C. Neurological involvement in HIV infection is more common in children than in adults. Neurological complications occur in > 40% of patients with HIV infection. They are the presenting feature of AIDS in 10–20% of patients. The prevalence of neuropathological abnormalities upon autopsy is 80%. Although an ongoing decline in HIV-associated CNS disease has been seen in very recent years, the mortality from these diseases remains elevated.

180.C.

181.B.   Serotonin is found in many cells that are not neurons, such as platelets, mast cells, and enterochromaffin cells. In fact, the brain accounts for only about 1% of body stores of serotonin.

182.E.   The alar plate gives rise to the layers of the superior colliculus and to the nuclei of the inferior colliculus.

183.A.   Studies comparing nucleus pulposus material from disk herniation versus painful degenerative disk disease have shown that protein expression of tumor necrosis factor-α (TNF-α) and interleukin (IL)-8 is increased in the degenerative disk disease group, and both groups had similar levels of IL-1β, IL-6, and IL-12. Therefore, TNF-α and IL-8 may be promising candidates to treat patients with diskogenic back pain on a molecular level.

184.D.   When dissecting below the arcuate line, the transversalis fascia is the only fascial layer between the rectus abdominis and the peritoneum.

185.B.   Cranial neuropathies are a more common presenting sign of ependymomas than other tumors due to their tendency to arise from the floor of the fourth ventricle. Medulloblastomas typically arise from the inferior medullary velum.

186.D.   Lissauer's tract caps the dorsal horns, and these fibers terminate in the substantia gelatinosa (lamina II).

187.B.   The limen insula is part of the primary olfactory cortex and is found at the junction of the insular and frontal lobe cortex.

188.C.   If the electrode is correctly placed, visual thresholds are usually between 2 and 3 V. Higher values indicate that the electrode is too far superior. Lower values indicate that the electrode is too far inferior.

189.C.

190.B.

191.B

192.A.   In stiff person syndrome, the stiffness primarily affects the truncal muscles and is superimposed by spasms, resulting in postural deformities. Chronic pain, impaired mobility, and lumbar hyperlordosis are common symptoms. The pattern of inheritance is unknown. Patients generally have high amounts of glutamic acid decarboxylase antibody titers.

193.B.   Inflammatory mediators including interleukin (IL)-1β, IL-6, IL-8, and tumor necrosis factor-α are expressed at higher levels in "diseased" intervertebral disks.

194.E.

195.A.

196.D. Enlarged pituitary stalk may be due to sarcoidosis, which can present with elevated angiotensin-converting enzyme levels. It may also be due to Langerhans cell histiocytosis, which may present with eosinophilic granuloma. It can occur in cases of meningitis in children. It is very rarely associated with primary pituitary tumors.

197.D. Central facial palsy is usually characterized by either hemiparalysis or hemiparesis of the contra-lateral muscles in facial expression. Muscles on the forehead are typically intact. Patients have lost voluntary control of muscle movement in the face; however, muscles in the face involved in spontaneous emotional expression usually remain intact.

198.C.

199.A. Esthesioneuroblastoma has a variable outcome that is primarily prognosticated by the extent of involvement at presentation (Kadish stage and lymph nodes metastasis) and completeness of resection.

200.E. Brainstem auditory evoked potentials (BSAEP) measure the timing of electrical waves from the brainstem in response to clicks or tone bursts in the ear. Computer averaging over time filters background noise to generate an averaged response of the auditory pathway to an auditory stimulus. Three waves (I, III and V) are plotted for each ear. The waveform represents specific anatomical points along the auditory neural pathway: the cochlear nerve and nuclei (waves I and II), superior olivary nucleus (wave III), lateral lemniscus (wave IV), and inferior colliculi (wave V). The most reliable indicator of retraction during vestibular schwannoma surgery from the BSAEP is the interaural latency differences in wave V; the latency in the abnormal ear is prolonged.

201.B.

202.E. Golgi tendon organs are sensitive to muscle tension.

203.D. Lyme disease is an inflammatory disease caused by the spirochetes Borrelia burgdorferi, which are transmitted by the bite of infected Ixodes ticks. Lyme disease is endemic in Massachusetts, Connecticut, Maine, New Hampshire, Rhode Island, New York, New Jersey, Pennsylvania, Delaware, Maryland, Michigan, and Wisconsin. It is categorized into early localized, early disseminated, and late. There may be an erythema migrans or systemic complaints in the early localized phase. Early disseminated Lyme disease can present with many central nervous system manifestations, including meningitis, altered mental status, radiculopathy and cranial neuropathy. If left untreated, sequelae include rheumatologic symptoms (monoarticular or oligoarticular arthritis) in 60%, neurologic signs and symptoms in 10%, and cardiac complications in 5% of cases.

204.A.   Shunt nephritis is a well-described complication of ventriculoatrial (VA) shunts. VA shunt complications are much more severe and potentially life-threatening than ventriculoperitoneal (VP) shunt complications.

205.C.   There is a paucity of mitoses and no necrosis in dysembryoplastic neuroepithelial tumors (DNET).

206.D.   The patient likely presents with an adrenocorticotropic hormone (ACTH)-secreting macroadenoma. Proper evaluation prior to surgery includes ophthalmologic and endocrine consultations and an endocrine panel of laboratory tests.

207.D.

208.D.   All of the information that is passed between the brainstem and the cerebellum enters and exits through one of three cerebellar peduncles: (1) inferior cerebellar peduncle or *restiform* body at the level of the medulla, (2) middle cerebellar peduncle or brachium pontis at the level of the pons, (3) superior cerebellar peduncle or brachium conjunctivum at the level of the midbrain. The vestibulocerebellar tract traverses the *juxtarestiform* body.

209.C.   Higher levels of TrkA are seen in neuroblastomas with favorable histology. The other factors listed are associated with a worse prognosis in neuroblastomas.

210.C.

211.C.   Choline acetyltransferase is the definitive marker for cholinergic neurons. Hemicholimium-3 blocks the high-affinity cholinergic reuptake process.

212.A.   Tanycytes are a variety of ependymal cells found in the wall of the third ventricle. The tanycyte is a cell with intermediate features between astrocytes and ependymal cells.

213.B.

214.D.

215.E.

216.C.   The diagram shown represents the lumbar plexus, structure A is the ilioinguinal nerve, B is the genitofemoral nerve, C is the lateral femoral cutaneous nerve, D is the femoral nerve, and E is the obturator nerve.

217.B.

218.B.   Facial agnosia (prosoprognosia) results from bilateral damage to the medial basal occipitotemporal cortex.

219.E.   All of the above may be the presentation in children with neuroblastomas. Diarrhea is from vasoactive intestinal polypeptide (VIP) secretion by the tumor. Ondine's curse results from impaired autonomic control of respiration.

220.C.

221.D.   The synthesis of NO (nitrous oxide) involves the conversion of L-arginine into NO and citrulline. All three isoforms of nitric oxide synthase (NOS) require tetrahydrobiopterin as a cofactor and NADPH as a coenzyme.

222.B.   The substantia gelatinosa (Rexed lamina II) is found at all cord levels and is homologous to the spinal trigeminal tract. It is associated with light touch, pain, and temperature sensation, and it integrates input for the ventral and lateral spinothalamic tracts.

223.A.   Vein of Galen malformation may be defined as a direct arteriovenous (AV) fistula between choroidal and/or quadrigeminal arteries and an overlying single median venous sac; it is rare, representing only < 1% of all intracranial arteriovenous malformations (AVMs). Neonatal patients present with an abrupt onset of high-output cardiac failure; as much as 80% of the cardiac output may pass through the fistula. An audible bruit may be present. Another type of vein of Galen malformation (VOGM) (presenting with ocular symptoms and developmental delay) is typically thalamic or midbrain with deep drainage to the vein of Galen (VOG).

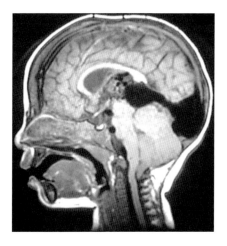

224.D.   The scan demonstrates an intramedullary cavernoma. These lesions tend to bleed in patients of young age, show a clear sensory level, present with subarachnoid hemorrhage or by progressive ascending paraplegic syndrome. The definitive therapy is microsurgical elimination.

225.B.   The arcuate eminence is a prominence on the anterior surface of the petrous portion of the temporal bone corresponding to the position of the superior semicircular canal.

226.D.

227.B.   The calamus scriptorius is an anatomic structure along the inferior part of the rhomboid fossa; the narrow lower end of the fourth ventricle between the two clavae.

228.D.   Delta waves occur with deep sleep, infancy, and brain disease.

229.E.   The stylohyoid is innervated by VII. The styloglossus is innervated by XII. The stylopharyngeus is innervated by IX.

230.A.   The sagittal vertical axis is the distance between the C7 plumb line and the posterosuperior corner of S1 in the sagittal plane.

231.A.   Allodynia is a condition in which a painful response is produced by an innocuous mechanical stimulation. It is the result of sensitization of spinothalamic neurons in the dorsal horn and the failure of descending systems to control the activity of these neurons. Alloesthesia is characterized by a painful stimulus on one side of the body that is thought to be on the other side.

232.D.   Clarke's nucleus is found at the base of the dorsal horn and corresponds to Rexed VII lamina. Clarke's column extends from C8 or T1 to about L3. Clarke's nucleus is homologous to the accessory cuneate nucleus of the medulla. It subserves unconscious proprioception from the muscle spindles and Golgi tendon organs and is the origin of the dorsal spinocerebellar tract.

233.E.   Basal encephaloceles should be treated as early as possible. Children with basal encephaloceles in the nasopharynx are at significant risk of developing meningitis.

234.B.   The anterior limb of the internal capsule (on horizontal section) can be found between the caudate nucleus and the corpus striatum (globus pallidus and putamen). Clinically important tracts lie in the genu and posterior limb. The posterior limb (on horizontal section) can be found between the thalamus and the corpus striatum (globus pallidus and putamen). The posterior limb of the internal capsule contains corticospinal fibers.

235.D.

236.A.

237.B.

238.C.

239.D. The greater occipital nerve is a sensory nerve from the dorsal ramus of C2.

240.C. Thromboxane synthesis inhibitors lead to a buildup of arachidonic acid.

241.C. The lateral portion of the substantia nigra pars reticulata (SNpr) is connected with cortical and brainstem areas that control eye movements. SNpr is GABAergic and inhibitory to the VLm (medial part of the ventrolateral thalamus) and VAmc (magnocellular part of the ventral anterior thalamus).

242.A. The dorsal lateral sulcus receives the dorsal roots.

243.D. The scan shows a diffusely enhancing brainstem glioma. Biopsy is usually not recommended in this case. Hyperfractionated radiation therapy has been shown to improve survival. Brainstem gliomas represent 10–20% of childhood CNS tumors. There are currently no proven chemotherapeutic regimens.

244.B. Pelvic incidence: the angle between the perpendicular to the sacral plate at its midpoint and the line connecting this point to the middle axis of the femoral heads. It is an anatomical parameter, unique to each individual, independent of the spatial orientation of the pelvis. Sacral slope: the angle between the superior plate of S1 and a horizontal line. Pelvic tilt: the angle between the line connecting the midpoint of the sacral plate to the axis of the femoral heads, and the vertical.

245.E. The MRI represents a midsagittal section demonstrating a large sellar and suprasellar mass that is compressing the optic chiasm. Slightly elevated prolactin level may be secondary to the stalk effect.

246.E.

247.D.

248.B. Lhermitte–Duclos disease is an uncommon cerebellar dysplasia that is characterized by hypertrophy of granular-cell neurons, and axonal hypermyelination in the molecular layer. Also known as dysplastic gangliocytoma of the cerebellum, it may occur in the setting of Cowden disease caused by a PTEN germline mutation.

249.A.   There is no sensory deficit and no decrease in corneal reflex. There are no other symptoms in the other cranial nerves.

250.B.   The liquid embolic agent n-butyl cyanoacrylate is used in interventional neuroradiology. The embolic agents that are particulate in nature include polyvinyl alcohol, platinum coils, and silk thread.

251.C.   The Glasgow Coma Scale score (GCS score) in this case would be 13. Eyes open to speech (3), the patient is confused (4), and he obeys motor commands (6)

252.B.   The ciliospinal center of Budge is found in the lateral horn at T1. This is a sympathetic nucleus that innervates the radial muscle of the iris (dilator pupillae) and the nonstriated superior and inferior (Müller) muscles.

253.E.   Aspirin decreases all anticonvulsant levels.

254.A.   Posterior inferior cerebellar artery (PICA) syndrome causes decreased contralateral pain and temperature of the body.

255.C.   Teardrop fractures occur when a fracture occurs on the anteroinferior edge of the vertebral body. The injury is due to hyperflexion and is unstable. Teardrop fractures are associated with anterior cord syndrome.

256.B.

257.B.   Dura and blood vessels are formed from mesoderm.

258.C.   The most common primary septal tumor is astrocytoma.

259.C.   The superior cerebellar artery is the most commonly conflicting artery in trigeminal neuralgia.

260.A.   The ELANA technique (excimer laser-assisted nonocclusive anastomosis) may be used to anastomose arteries.

261.B.   This MRI scan demonstrates a unilateral jumped facet with rotation in the cervical cord, compromising the spinal canal.

262.D.   This particular AVM is best-graded 4A. Its medium size (2), eloquent location (1), and deep drainage (1) place it as a Spetzler–Martin grade 4. The fact that it has stenotic venous drainage gives it a subclassification of 4A.

263.B. Biot (irregular breathing) is caused by a lesion in the dorsomedial medulla.

264.B. The anterior choroidal artery supplies the internal globus pallidus, posterior limb of the internal capsule, and temporal horn of the choroid plexus.

265.D. Pronator teres syndrome is different from carpal tunnel syndrome in that patients with pronator teres syndrome exhibit numbness in the palm, and nocturnal exacerbations are rare.

266.C. The MRI scan represents a brain midsagittal section demonstrating descent of the cerebellar vermis or tonsils consistent with a Chiari malformation, given the age of the patient and the absence of other findings (e.g., hydrocephalus or medullary kinking), this most likely represents a Chiari type 1 malformation.

267.C.

268.B.

269.B. Although it is true that the pain starts at V_2 (the lower side of the nose) and then involves V_3 and V_1, it is only necessary to treat the trigger zone.

270.E. Gerstmann's syndrome is caused by a dominant parietal lobe lesion (angular gyrus) and includes agraphia without alexia (patient can read but cannot write). Astereognosis is also caused by dominant parietal lobe lesions but is not part of Gerstmann's syndrome.

271.E. Epidermoids of the skull show a lytic defect with a scalloped, sclerotic rim. They are slow growing and rarely show malignant transformation.

272.E.

273.B. Nightmares occur during REM sleep; night terrors may occur in either stage 3 or 4 sleep. Stage 4 sleep is associated with delta waves.

274.A.
275.D.

276.B. A high-riding jugular bulb may be encountered during the drilling portion and should be tamponaded with hemostatic products and cottonoids.

277.B.   The subcommissural organ is the only circumventricular organ with an intact blood–brain barrier (BBB).

278.B.   Dysgeusias are particularly prevalent in the elderly and are often associated with the use of antihypertensives (e.g., captopril).

279.C.   Gamma knife treatment is the best mode of therapy for an AVM that is smaller than 3 cm and located in an eloquent area. The angiogram shows a small subcortical right parietal arteriovenous malformation with filling vessel arising from a branch of the right middle cerebral artery. Venous drainage is noted into the upper sagittal sinus.

280.D.   Foster–Kennedy syndrome is usually caused by an olfactory groove or medial-third sphenoid wing tumor (usually meningioma). The classic triad is anosmia (ipsilateral), central scotoma (ipsilateral), and papilledema (contralateral).

281.B.   Pick's disease is characterized by severe focal atrophy commonly in the frontal and temporal lobes. This results in mental status and personality changes occurring in Pick's patients. Pick bodies are positive for *tau* protein.

282.B.   Fibrillation potentials are triphasic and last 1–5 ms caused by the activity of one fiber.

283.B.   Sleep spindles (the burst described) and K complexes (sharp slow waves of high amplitude) are characteristic of stage 2 sleep.

284.D.   The bony promontory seen in the picture is the posterior clinoid process and may be drilled carefully to expose the neck of the aneurysm.

285.D.   The suprascapular nerve is trapped in the suprascapular notch. This nerve is the branch of the superior trunk. Atrophy of the supraspinatus and infraspinatus can result.

286.C.   The abducens nerve crosses the medial lemniscus on exiting the brainstem.

287.B.   The correct units are 50 mL/100 g/min.

288.D.

289.A.   Removal of frontal meningiomas may improve attentional functions. There are minimal differences in memory, visuoconstructive abilities, or executive functions.

290.E. The secretion of prolactin by lactotroph cells is inhibited by dopamine released by hypothalamic neurons.

291.C. The substantia nigra pars reticulata neurons related to saccadic eye movements decrease their activity during the saccade.

292.D.

293.A. Research with model systems of seemingly disparate species (i.e., marine snail and albino rat) suggest that neural mechanisms involved in associative learning may be highly conserved across species.

294.E.

295.C. Hypothermia is characterized by J-point elevation.

296.A. Anterior encephaloceles are compatible with normal intelligence in the majority of patients. Atretic encephaloceles also appear not to influence intellectual development and also have a low incidence of hydrocephalus.

297.A. Giant cell glioblastoma is shown in the slide. The hallmark of giant cell glioblastoma is predominance on multinucleated giant cells and a high frequency of the TP53 mutation.

298.D. These features should not necessarily prompt the diagnosis of glioblastoma.

299.B. The supramarginal gyrus is at the posterior reach of the sylvian fissure.

300.A. Avellis's syndrome is caused by a brainstem lesion that limits vagal innervation unilaterally, resulting in ipsilateral paralysis of the vocal cord and soft palate and loss of sensitivity to pain and temperature in the contralateral leg, trunk, arm, and neck. This syndrome is also called ambiguospinothalamic paralysis.

301.E. Bicuculline is a GABA-A antagonist. Muscimol is a GABA-A agonist. Kynurenate is a glutamate antagonist. Picrotoxin is a GABA inhibitor.

302.B. There is increased production of PMP22 in Charcot–Marie–Tooth disease.

303.C. Neurons in the spinal nucleus and in the ventral parts of the chief sensory nucleus give rise to the crossed ventral trigeminothalamic tract.

304.D.   In stroboscopic illumination at flicker rates below 15 Hz, the motion system is disabled. This explains why nightclub dancers are seen as moving discontinuously under a strobe light.

305.C.   The tectospinal tract decussates in the dorsal tegmental decussation. Tectospinal fibers originate from deeper layers of the superior colliculus and distribute to cervical cord levels. Rubrospinal fibers decussate in the ventral tegmental decussation.

306.A.   In the Royal Melbourne Hospital series of paranasal sinus involvement treated by craniofacial resection, sphenoid sinus involvement was the major predictor of later tumor recurrence.

307.E.   Bipolar cells serve as interneurons between photoreceptor cells and ganglion cells.

308.D.

309.B.

310.C.   The connatal form (type II) is clinically more severe and symptoms begin in the neonatal period. Pelizaeus–Merzbacher disease (PMD) results from mutations affecting the gene for proteolipid protein (PLP).

311.D.   The pontocerebellar tract passes to the cerebellum via the middle cerebellar peduncle. The ventral spinocerebellar tract and the tectocerebellar tract pass through the superior cerebellar peduncle.

312.C.   The lateral zone (dentate) sends fibers to the VL thalamus and motor cortex (area 4). A lesion of the anterior lobe may cause slight hyperreflexia.

313.A.   Dendrodendritic synapses have been found in the olfactory bulb and have been shown to be inhibitory; the granule cells processes make synaptic contacts with dendrites of mitral cells. Axodendritic synapses are excitatory. Axosomatic synapses are inhibitory, and a classic example is the cerebellar basket cell contacting the Purkinje cell.

314.B.   The parvocellular system of the dorsal lateral geniculate nucleus makes up about 80% of the total ganglion cell number.

315.E.   During a neurosurgical procedure, a sudden decrease in end tidal CO_2 suggests venous air embolus and may even precede the appreciation of changes by the precordial Doppler.

316.E.   These structures run in the floor of the body of the lateral ventricle.

317.A.   The contents of the cubital fossa from medial to lateral are the median nerve, brachial artery, biceps brachii tendon, and radial nerve.

318.D.   The teres minor rotates the arm laterally.

319.C.   The internal cerebral vein position can be confirmed by superimposing the angiogram of the medial posterior choroidal artery with the venous phase. The internal cerebral vein and the medial posterior choroidal artery occupy the same position when the arterial and venous phase are superimposed. Both of these structures course within the cistern of the velum interpositum.

320.B.

321.D.   The Botzinger complex is the principle source of reciprocal inhibition in the respiratory network. It comprises a cluster of cells at the rostral-most tip of the ventral respiratory group.

322.D.   The posterior cord gives rise to the upper subscapular, lower subscapular, and thoracodorsal nerves. The latissimus dorsi is innervated by the thoracodorsal nerve. The subscapularis muscle is innervated by the upper and lower sub-scapular nerve. The teres major is innervated by the lower subscapular nerve.

323.A.   The vast majority of children present with ischemic symptoms (transient ischemic attacks (TIAs), extremity weakness), whereas adults typically present with hemorrhage.

324.C.   Valproic acid has a short half-life (~ 8 hours). Association with platelet dysfunction should alert the surgeon to the possibility of bleeding problems, especially in epilepsy cases.

325.B.   Isoflurane allows patients to emerge from anesthesia faster, and there is less hepatic effect from this agent. In addition, isoflurane produces the least increase in cerebral blood flow (CBF) of inhalational anesthetics.

326.C.   The glomus is a prominent tuft of choroid plexus found in the atrium.

327.C.   The axillary nerve passes posteriorly around the surgical neck of the humerus. The radial nerve lies in the radial groove of the middle of the shaft of the humerus. The ulnar nerve passes behind the medial epicondyle. All three of these nerves are susceptible to humerus fractures since they lie in close contact with bone.

328.C.   The premotor area plays a role in programming and sequencing learned complex movements.

329.E.

330.A.   Theta activity has a frequency of 4–7 Hz. Other common electroencephalographic (EEG) rhythms are delta (0–3 Hz), alpha (8–13 Hz), and beta (> 13 Hz).

331.B.   The mesencephalic nucleus of the trigeminal nerve has pseudounipolar neurons. The mesencephalic nucleus extends from the pons to the upper midbrain. It receives input from muscle spindles and pressure receptors.

332.B.   These second-order neurons will give rise to axons that enter the cerebellum via the superior cerebellar peduncle. The ventral spinocerebellar tract conveys efference copies of motor commands for the lower extremities.

333.B.   Chromophobic cells lack cytoplasmic granules. They represent acidophil or basophil cells after the release of hormone-containing granules. They have no stain reaction after PAS stain.

334.D.   The extent of mesiobasal resection determines the outcome after temporal lobectomy for intractable complex partial seizures.

335.E.   Sydenham's chorea is the most common type of chorea. Also known as St. Vitus's dance, this chorea occurs mainly in young females after a bout of rheumatic fever.

336.D.   This is decadron. A postoperative course of an H2-receptor blocker is indicated for patients on glucocorticoid treatment.

337.D.

338.B.   Ventralis intermedius (Vim) stimulation is the procedure of choice when contralateral thalamotomy has been performed or is anticipated.

339.C.   Temozolomide (TMZ) is an orally administered chemotherapeutic (alkyl-ating) agent with minimal side effects that readily crosses the blood–brain barrier and is approved for treating anaplastic astrocytomas.

340.D.   The H-reflex is a submaximal stimulation of mixed motor-sensory nerves, not enough to cause a direct motor response. The H-reflex is the electrical representation of the tendon reflex circuit.

341.B.   The most common and pronounced aging effect on the brain is cell loss.

342.A.   Stereognosis is an important function of the dorsal column–medial lemnis-cal system.

343.C.   Irrigation of fluid-coupled monitoring systems increases the infection rate nearly threefold. Thus irrigation, if necessary, should be performed infrequently and with exquisite sterile technique.

344.E.   Area 4 fibers terminate in laminae VI–IX, whereas fibers starting in laminae IV and V project to the postcentral gyrus via the spino-thalamic tract. The anterior corticospinal tract is an uncrossed tract in the (medial) ventral cord and terminates on lamina VII.

345.E.   The paracentral lobule is supplied by branches from the anterior cerebral artery.

346.D.

347.D.

348.D.   The sensorimotor GPi is located in the posterolateral part of the nucleus.

349.A.   The lesion represents a nerve root schwannoma. The majority of these arise from a dorsal nerve root. Ten to 15% extend through the dural root sleeve. The fourth through sixth decades represent the peak incidence of occurrence. Schwannomas are typically described as smooth globoid and do not produce enlargement of the nerve but are suspended eccentrically from it with a discrete attachment.

350.D.   Type I fibers are characterized by slow contraction times and a high resistance to fatigue. Structurally, they have a small motor neuron and fiber diameter, a high mitochondrial and capillary density, and a high myoglobin content.

351.C.   Cowdry type A inclusions are intranuclear and are seen with cytomegalovirus, herpes, and subacute sclerosing panencephalitis (SSPE). Cowdry type B inclusions are intranuclear and are seen in acute poliovirus. The others listed are intracytoplasmic inclusions. Lafora bodies are seen in myoclonic epilepsy. Bunina bodies are seen in amyotrophic lateral sclerosis (ALS).

352.D.   The dorsal spinocerebellar is an uncrossed tract.

353.D.   Nystagmus in Ménière's disease is horizontal and contralateral to the affected side. Past-pointing and falling occur toward the affected side.

354.A.   The pulvinar has reciprocal connections with the inferior parietal lobule.

355.E.

356.B.   Pineal tumors usually lie between the precentral cerebellar vein and the vein of Galen. The precentral cerebellar vein is usually displaced posterosuperiorly. This vein may be sacrificed if necessary.

357.C.   The pharyngeal tubercle is found in line with the vomer and foramen magnum at the cranial base.

358.D.   The anterior choroidal and lateral posterior choroidal supply the lateral ventricle. The medial posterior choroidal supplies the choroid plexus of the third ventricle. The posterior inferior cerebellar artery (PICA) supplies the choroid plexus of the third ventricle.

359.E.   The liver damage causes the levels of ammonia to rise because it is not converted to urea; this may lead to increased production of GABA. Glutamate is not involved.

360.D. Wilson's disease (hepatolenticular degeneration) is a familial metabolic disease transmitted as an autosomal recessive trait. The abnormal gene has been assigned to the esterase D locus on chromosome 13.

361.B. Bergmann glia have cell bodies located in the Purkinje layer of the cerebellar cortex.

362.E. This is a lower motor neuron lesion and Babinski's sign would not be expected.

363.C. The static labyrinth consists of the utricle and saccule. The vestibule is a central cavity of the inner ear that contains the saccule and utricle.

364.D. The ventral posteromedial (VPM) nucleus receives taste input via the ipsilateral central tegmental tract. The VPM nucleus receives sensory input from the head and oral cavity.

365.A. The lateral suboccipital retrosigmoid approach is best used for lateral tentorial notch meningiomas that extend infratentorially.

366.A. Calcifications are likely to be abnormal if encountered in children younger than 6 years. The incidence of pineal calcification is at most 40% by the age of 18.

367.E. The anterior longitudinal ligament attaches the dens to the anterior tubercle of the atlas. The transverse ligament of the atlas is posterior to the dens. The apical and alar ligaments attach the dens to the foramen magnum.

368.B. The most frequent site of subependymoma is the fourth ventricle (50–60% of cases), followed by the lateral ventricles (30–40%). Less common sites are the third ventricle and septum pellucidum.

369.C. The lamina terminalis fills the interval between the anterior commissure and the optic chiasm.

370.A. Damage to the right frontal eye field (area 8) results in deviation of the eyes to the right.

371.D. Choroid plexus papillomas frequently display immunopositivity for transthyretin (prealbumin) and S-100.

372.B. Between 15 and 20 mL/100 g/min cortical evoked responses are lost and the (EEG) becomes isoelectric, but the neurons remain viable and are described as "idling." At about 30 mL/100 g/min, the patient loses consciousness.

373.C. The lateral vestibulospinal tract is an uncrossed tract.

374.E. Lesions of the mediodorsal nucleus are found in patients with the Korsakoff amnestic state.

375.B. The trochlear nerve should be identified before transecting the tentorium.

376.C. Germinomas commonly occur in males in the first 3 decades.

377.D. Pathologically central nervous system (CNS) sarcoid is characterized by non-caseating granulomas.

378.A. Although other tumors may be more common after 1 year of life, choroid plexus tumors are the most common tumor in the first year of life.

379.B. A "square" ACA shift is usually caused by a holotemporal mass.

380.D.

381.A. The obex is the caudal apex of the rhomboid fossa and marks the beginning of the "open medulla."

382.B. Hyponatremia (Na < 130) can occur in up to 30% of ruptured anterior communicating artery aneurysms due to the local proximity of key perforators that supply the anterior hypothalamic nuclei.

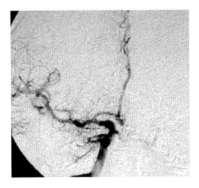

383.C.

384.E. The optic disc (optic papilla) is located 3.5 mm nasal to the fovea centralis. It contains unmyelinated axons from the ganglion cell layer of the retina. The optic disc is the blind spot (contains neither rods nor cones).

385.C. The inferior obliquus capitis muscle forms a common border of the superior and inferior suboccipital triangles. The lateral borders of both triangles meet at the transverse process of the atlas, which is located 1 cm below the mastoid tip.

386.C. The facial nerve needs to be identified medially close to the brain stem and followed laterally.

387.C. Plain film calcification is rarely seen. Calcospheres are also known as psammoma bodies.

388.E. The infraspinatus is innervated by the suprascapular nerve, which originates from the upper trunk of the brachial plexus. The subscapularis is innervated by the upper and lower subscapular nerves. The teres major is innervated by the lower subscapular nerve. The latissimus dorsi is innervated by the thoracodorsal nerve. The teres minor is innervated by the axillary nerve.

389.C. The time of development of effects of radiation is dose independent.

390.E. Mitochondrial encephalomyopathy, lactic acidosis, and stroke-like episodes (MELAS) is a condition that affects many of the body's systems, particularly the brain and nervous system (encephalo-) and muscles (myopathy). MERRF stands for "myoclonic epilepsy with ragged-red fibers." Kawasaki disease is a condition that causes inflammation in the walls of medium-sized arteries throughout the body, including the coronary arteries, which supply blood to the heart muscle. Kawasaki disease is also called mucocutaneous lymph node syndrome because it also affects lymph nodes, skin, and the mucous membranes inside the mouth, nose and throat. The etiology of Kawasaki disease is unknown. Most of the epidemiologic and immunologic evidence indicates that the causative agent is probably infectious. However, autoimmune reactions and genetic predisposition are suggested as possible etiologic factors.

391.E. Amplification of epidermal growth factor (EGF) occurs in glioblastoma. Double minutes (cytogenetic evidence of gene amplification) of N-myc occurs in medulloblastoma.

392.A. The Goldman cardiac risk score for noncardiac surgery indicates that a recent myocardial infarction (MI) is a contraindication to elective surgery.

393.C. The fastigiovestibular tract is an efferent pathway that passes through the superior cerebellar peduncle (SCP) (uncinate fasciculus of the SCP). The juxtarestiform body is a component of the inferior cerebellar peduncle and contains afferent (vestibulocerebellar) and efferent (cerebellovestibular) fibers.

394.B. Bilateral destruction of both cunei results in a lower altitudinal hemianopia.

395.E. A posterior communicating artery aneurysm is prone to rupture with retraction on the temporal lobe.

396.B. Wave 5 is an indication of auditory nerve activity central to the tumor. It is easier to detect than the other waves. Wave 5 is generated in the brainstem. When used with N1 (monitors action potential of the auditory nerve), it is useful for predicting postoperative hearing function.

397.D. The most common symptom at initial presentation is referable to sensation.

398.E. The dorsomedial thalamus is a part of the basolateral circuit. The basolateral circuit passes from the orbitofrontal cortex to the anterior temporal cortex via the uncinate fasciculus, then to the amygdala and the dorsomedial nucleus of the thalamus, and back to the orbitofrontal cortex via a thalamofrontal radiation. The circuit of Papez passes from the septal region via the cingulated bundle to the hippocampus, then via the fornix to the mammillary bodies via the mammillothalamic tract to the anterior thalamus, then from the anterior thalamus back to the cingulum.

399.A. White matter degeneration of the subcortical U-fibers. This is a feature of Canavan's disease, which is a different metabolic disease with the same inheritance pattern and is caused by a deficiency of the enzyme N-acetyl-aspartoacylase.

400.E. Broca's aphasia results from damage to Brodmann area 44 (inferior frontal gyrus). The most common cause of expressive aphasia is stroke. The most effective pharmacological treatments are piracetam and amphetamine.

401.B. Canavan's disease is associated with a point mutation of aspartoacylase 2 leading to elevated levels of N-acetylaspartic acid (NAA). It is a progressive, fatal neurological disorder that is caused by this mutation, which affects myelin.

402.C. Antiplatelet drugs are the most common cause of platelet disorders leading to excessive bleeding at surgery. Excessive bleeding in surgery can usually be seen early at skin incision and during initial dissection. If the surgeon believes that the unexpected excessive bleeding will pose a risk to the patient, it is advisable to abort the procedure, obtain a hematology consult, and proceed with surgery on another day. If the surgeon decides that the bleeding is not going to pose a threat to the patient, it is advisable to leave a small drain under only light bulb suction (not fully compressed suction), to use a pressure dressing at the end of the case, and to obtain a hematocrit after the case.

403.A. Poxvirus is a DNA virus. Viral meningitis occurs in up to 50% of paramyx-ovirus infections (mumps). Rabies (rhabdovirus) targets the limbic tissue. DNA viruses cause SSPE, PML (papovavirus), and herpes encephalitis. RNA viruses are implicated in meningitis, AIDS, Ebola, severe acute respiratory syndrome (SARS), West Nile, and polio. Herpes simplex encephalitis (HSE) is the only CNS viral infection whose course and outcome are improved by specific antiviral therapy (acyclovir). HSE can lie dormant in the ganglion of the trigeminal nerve causing trigeminal neuralgia. If acyclovir is not helpful, radiosurgical treatment of the trigeminal nerve may be indicated.

404.D. Hematoporphyrin derivative is an agent that is capable of photosensitizing malignant tumor cells. Other photosensitizers include rhodamine, acridine orange, phthalocyanines, and pyrilium derivatives.

405.B. The cranial nerve most sensitive to radiation is the optic nerve and the chi-asm, with a single fraction dose tolerance of 8 Gy. Other cranial nerves can be affected from radiation in order of frequency: XII, XI, X, V, and VI. The recurrent laryngeal nerve can be injured after radiation therapy for breast or lung cancers; therefore, in anterior cervical discectomy and fusion (ACDF) cases, patients with a history of radiation in these areas should be briefed on the higher risk of hoarseness and vocal changes after surgery.

406.A. The junction of the transverse and sigmoid sinuses is usually located 1–1.5 cm rostral to the mastoid emissary vein. In this photograph (reprinted with permission from The American Society of Neuroradiology) the mastoid emissary vein is labeled *n*, the transverse sinus is labeled *b*, and the sigmoid sinus is labeled *c*. Profuse bleeding can be seen in dissections near this vein as well as other veins in the cerebellar area. It is important for the surgeon to have hemoclips, hemostatic packing agents, and BioGlue (CryoLife)/DuraSeal (Optimus Medical) ready in the room should the need arise in any posterior fossa surgery.

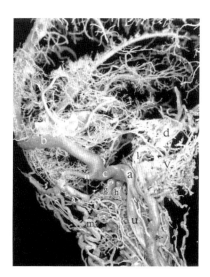

407.B. The Rexed laminae is the system of ten layers of gray matter (I–X) named after Swedish neuroscientist Bror Rexed in the 1950s. (Figure from THIEME Atlas of Anatomy, Head and Neuroanatomy, © Thieme 2007, Illustration by Markus Voll.)

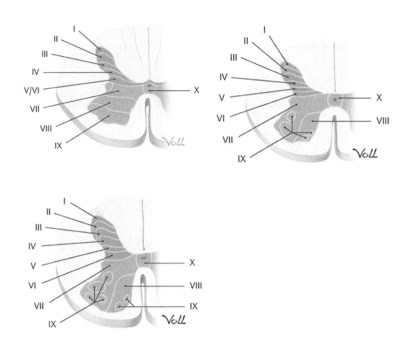

408.D. Cerebellar glomeruli are small, intertwined nerve fiber terminals in the granular layer of the cerebellar cortex. Glomeruli contain synaptic connections that contain axons of incoming mossy fibers, axons and dendrites of Golgi type II cells, and dendrites of granule cells. Purkinje cells are not part of the glomerulus. The cerebellar glomeruli are the first stop for afferent nerve fibers entering the cerebellum.

409.E. Focal white matter necrosis is the most common histological evidence of late radiation-related CNS injury.

410.D. Sacral. The gray matter changes shape throughout the spinal cord depending on the neural requirements of a given region.

411.B. Cerebral autosomal dominant arteriopathy with subcortical infarcts (CA-DASIL) leads to subcortical ischemic damage, myelin loss, lacunar infarcts, and gliosis. Ischemic strokes are the most frequent presentation of CADASIL where the underlying pathology is progressive degeneration of the smooth muscles cells in blood vessels.

412.C. Exacerbation of peptic ulcer is the most common side effect of high-dose dexamethasone. A short course (e.g., ≤ 4 days) of steroids does not need to be tapered. Longer courses of steroids should be tapered gradually.

413.A. Headache is almost universally noted in patients with cryptococcal meningitis. Poor prognosis of cryptococcal meningitis is seen with positive India ink stain, low CSF leukocyte count, a positive blood culture, presence of *C. neoformans* at extraneural sites, high CSF cryptococcal antigen titers, CSF hypoglycorrhachia, and an increased CSF opening pressure. Pharmacological treatment involves amphotericin B plus flucytosine.

414.E. Since over 85% of cerebrospinal fluid leaks from basilar skull fractures will resolve spontaneously, the primary approach is expectant observation. Prophylactic antibiotics have not been shown to decrease the risk of meningitis and are not recommended. CSF diversion with lumboperitoneal shunts may be used for refractory cases.

415.C. Pituitary tumors that secrete thyroid-stimulating hormone (TSH) also frequently co-secrete the glycoprotein hormone alpha-subunit. An alpha-subunit:TSH ratio of > 1 favors the diagnosis of TSH-secreting adenoma. TSH is a glycoprotein and consists of two subunits, alpha and beta. The alpha subunit is identical to that of human chorionic gonadotropin (hCG), luteinizing hormone (LH), and follicle-stimulating hormone (FSH). The beta subunit is unique to TSH and determines its receptor specificity.

416.A. The superior (anterior) semicircular canal is identified by the arcuate eminence at the base of the skull.

417.D. The inferior orbital fissure is formed by the orbital surface of the greater wing of the sphenoid and the orbital surface of the maxilla. The inferior division of the ophthalmic vein passes through the inferior orbital fissure.

418.A.   Many spinocerebellar fibers are distributed to the medial vermal region of the anterior lobe of the cerebellum.

419.E.   Aneurysms are not indications for radiosurgery. The prevalence of intracranial aneurysm is about 1–5% so observation may be indicated in the majority of healthy patients where small aneurysms are found incidentally.

420.C.   The lesion is an epidermoid of the cerebellopontine angle. Epidermoid usually presents in the 20- to 40-year age group. Unlike dermoids, they are not associated with midline defect. Spilling of their contents may cause a chemical meningitis or ventriculitis; therefore spillage of tumor contents in the subarachnoid space must be avoided. The main goal of therapy is complete excision of the tumor wall and contents to prevent recurrences. Radiation or chemotherapy has no role in the management. Steroids have been shown to be effective in preventing the inflammatory response and possible ventriculitis associated with these tumors.

421.B.   Adrenoleukodystrophy displays X-linked recessive inheritance. Maple syrup urine disease is an autosomal recessive metabolic disorder affecting branched-chain amino acids. Adrenoleukodystrophy is a disorder of peroxisomal fatty acid beta oxidation, which results in accumulation of very-long-chain fatty acids. Wilson's disease is an autosomal recessive disorder where there is an alteration of the ATP7B gene resulting in inability to excrete copper from the body. Refsum's disease is an autosomal recessive neurological disease that results from overaccumulation of phytanic acid in cells and tissues. Homocystinuria is an inherited disorder of the metabolism of the amino acid methionine.

422.D.   In cerebral salt wasting syndrome (CSWS), there is inappropriate natriuresis and diuresis. CSWS is an endocrine condition of low sodium and dehydration in response to trauma, intracranial hematoma, or the presence of brain tumors.

423.D.   The presenting neurological symptoms and signs in HIV-infected individuals with *Toxoplasma* encephalitis are focal in nature. Hemiparesis is the most common focal finding.

424.D.   The fracture that initiates the leptomeningeal cyst may not be clinically evident but most commonly involves the parietal bone. A growing fracture can occur anywhere, including the skull base. Skull radiographs and CT scans are useful at initial injury and at follow-up.

425.C. Octreotide is fairly well tolerated; however, gallstone formation can develop in 10–20% of patients and is related to the inhibitory effect of octreotide on gallbladder motility. Other adverse effects of octreotide are headache, hypothyroidism, cardiac conduction abnormalities, and gastrointestinal reactions.

426.D. Stereotactic radiosurgery is becoming the standard of care for acoustic neuromas. The need for a tissue biopsy (which adds additional risk) is becoming less important in these tumors because radiological features are usually all that is needed to start treatment. In the event that one is mistaken and a meningioma is truly in the cerebellopontine (CP) angle, the radiosurgical dosage is essentially the same. Tissue diagnoses are especially dangerous in intramedullary spinal cord tumors where the patient is neurologically intact. Empirical radiosurgery performed on spinal cord tumors is being reported to have good results.

427.A. Bill's bar is named after William Fouts House (1923–2012), an American otologist referred to as Dr. Bill. This landmark divides the superior compartment of the internal acoustic meatus into an anterior and posterior compartment. Anterior to Bill's bar, in the anterior superior quadrant, are the facial nerve and nervus intermedius, and posterior to it in the posterior superior quadrant is the superior division of the vestibular nerve.

428.E. The fetal posterior communicating (Pcom) artery is the most frequent of the persistent fetal circulations. PCom aneurysms are one of the most common aneurysms, accounting for 25% of intracranial aneurysms. These aneurysms are often associated with large or fetal PCom arteries, and the treatment of these aneurysms requires significant diligence in order to maintain flow in the PCom artery.

429.D. An acoustic neuroma is shown in the radiograph and angiography has no role in the management of acoustic tumor.

430.D. Interruption of Meyer's loop fibers in the temporal lobe results in the "pie in the sky" lesion.

431.C. CAG is a common trinucleotide repeat and is translated into a series of uninterrupted glutamine residues forming a polyglutamine tract.

432.C.

433.A.   If a motor task is performed repeatedly to mastery, there is progressive attenuation of the cerebellar and premotor areas, with no change of activity of the primary motor cortex. This can be verified with fMRI scanning.

434.B.   The classic lucid interval is seen in only one-third of patients. Traction on the greater superficial petrosal nerve may occur with traction on the floor of the middle fossa, which may result in a dry eye postoperatively. Tacking sutures at surgery may be used for tenting of the dura during healing; however, a small, round JP drain with small holes under bulb suction for a couple days can work just as well, especially in a young patient.

435.D.   All are indications for craniotomy. Pituitary tumors can be effectively debulked with their remnant treated with radiosurgery several months later.

436.C.   An ABI (auditory brainstem implant) is designed to stimulate auditory neurons of the cochlear nucleus and is placed in the lateral recess of the fourth ventricle at the time of acoustic tumor removal.

437.A.   The dorsal scapular nerve arises from the brachial plexus, usually from the plexus root of C5. This nerve leaves C5 and commonly pierces the middle scalene muscle and continues deep to the levator scapulae and the rhomboids.

438.E.   All are associated with neurofibrillary tangles. Neurofibrillary tangles are the results of defective assembly of microtubules and/or neurofilaments. These tangles are aggregates of hyperphosphorylated tau proteins.

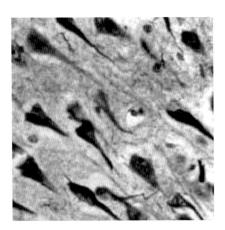

439.E.   The gyrus rectus may be removed (medial to olfactory nerve) in order to gain better visualization before clipping of an anterior communicating artery aneurysm.

440.C.   At the optic strut, the ophthalmic artery pierces the dura to enter the orbit. After the origin of the ophthalmic artery, the ICA passes the tip of the anterior clinoid process.

441.D.   *Cuneus* is Latin for *wedge*. The cuneus corresponds to Brodmann area 17 and is a smaller lobe in the occipital lobe of the brain. It is involved in basic visual processing.

442.B.   The size of the hematoma is inversely related to the chance of the patient developing vasospasm. This reflects the fact that most of the blood has gone into the brain rather than the subarachnoid space.

443.A.   Volatile anesthetics produce a dose-related reduction in CMR and a simultaneous increase in CBF. Intravenous anesthetic agents (except ketamine) decrease CMR and CBF in parallel. Volatile anesthetic agents increase CSF production.

444.E.   Note that the median sensory response, mediated by upper trunk fibers, would remain normal in lower trunk plexopathy. Trauma accounts for the majority of brachial plexus plexopathies. A lesion of the brachial plexus can result in motor, sensory, and sympathetic findings.

445.D.   An abnormal skin histamine response is a characteristic feature of patients with familial dysautonomia. Familial dysautonomia is also called Riley–Day syndrome and hereditary sensory and autonomic neuropathy type III. Familial dysautonomia is seen almost exclusively in Ashkenazi Jews and is inherited in an autosomal recessive fashion.

446.C.   The jugular foramen transmits a number of vital structures from the posterior fossa to the neck. This foramen is situated at the junction of the temporal and occipital bone. It is the site for glomus jugulare tumors, schwannomas, and meningiomas. Glomus tumors produce local bony destruction, whereas schwannomas produce a smooth-edged enlargement of the foramen.

447.B.   Acetylcholine and substance P are transmitters in this projection. The fasciculus retroflexus is also known as the habenulointerpeduncular tract. The habenula receives input from the brain via the stria medullaris thalami and outputs to many midbrain areas involved in releasing neurotransmitters such as dopamine, norepinephrine, and serotonin.

448.B. Charcot–Bouchard aneurysms (also known as military aneurysms or microaneurysms) are aneurysms of the brain vasculature that occur in small blood vessels < 300 µm diameter. They are most often located in the lenticulostriate vessels of the basal ganglia and are associated with chronic hypertension.

449.D. The lesion is a cavernous sinus meningioma. Lesions in this region that are approximately ≤ 3 cm are ideal for radiosurgery.

450.C. The anterior inferior cerebellar artery loops around cranial nerves VII and VIII.

451.D. The facial colliculus is located in the pontine half of the rhomboid fossa. The tuberculum cinereum (not to be confused with the tuber cinereum of the hypothalamus) is a surface eminence of the medulla that overlies the spinal trigeminal tract and nucleus.

452.C. Hemosiderin-laden macrophages are seen with cavernous malformation.

453.C. Calcium channel–blocking agents can be expected to have a beneficial effect in the patient; however, there is no lasting effect on angiographic vasospasm and no increase in CBF. The evidence for calcium channel blocking agents is not beyond all doubt, but given the potential benefits and modest risks of this treatment, it is indicated in patients with aneurysmal SAH.

454.D. The top of the cranial loop is the choroidal point, located in the telovelotonsillar segment of the PICA. The plexal point is the point where the anterior choroidal artery enters the choroidal fissure.

455.B. The principal anatomical substrate of perceptual organization is the posterior right hemisphere. Posterior right hemisphere lesions tend to produce the most severe deficits of constructional praxis.

456.A. Trautman's triangle is a space bounded by bony labyrinth anteriorly, sigmoid sinus posteriorly, and dura containing superior petrosal sinus superiorly. This area is a route where infections of temporal bone may traverse and affect the cerebellum.

457.B. The lateral lemniscus is a tract of axons in the brainstem that carries information about sound from the cochlear nucleus to various brainstem nuclei and ultimately the contralateral inferior colliculus of the midbrain.

458.D. These tumors are rare, but they must enter into the differential diagnosis of a solid third ventricle enhancing mass that is glial fibrillary acidic protein (GFAP) positive.

459.C. Impending herniation regardless of the tumor size or number is an indication for open surgery. One can proceed empirically with cranial radiosurgery without tissue biopsy with good results. A short course of steroids after radiosurgery is indicated for swelling prophylaxis.

460.B. The sphenoparietal sinus runs along the ridge of the sphenoid lesser wing and collects tributaries of the sylvian veins to empty into the cavernous sinus.

461.E. The precuneus is bounded posteriorly by the parieto-occipital sulcus. This area is involved with self-consciousness, memory, and visual-spatial processing.

462.B. Venous malformations may occur in up to 2% of individuals. Venous vascular malformations are also known as venous angiomas. A newer term, *developmental venous anomalies (DVA)*, has been recommended as a more appropriate term.

463.A. The anterior meningeal artery is also known as the anterior falx artery. This artery can be enlarged in frontal tumors, falcine meningiomas, and moyamoya disease.

464.C. The recurrent artery of Heubner enters the anterior perforating substance and supplies the head of the caudate, anterior limb of the internal capsule, the anterior putamen and GP, the septal nuclei, and the inferior frontal lobe. Otto Heubner was a German pediatrician who made contributions in cerebrospinal meningitis, syphilitic endarteritis obliterans, aseptic practices in the hospital environment, and infectious disease.

465.C. The external sphincter is composed of circularly arranged striated muscle fibers that are mostly type I (slow twitch).

466.D. Harris's method is the most clinically useful means of assessing atlanto-occipital dislocation. The basion should lie within 12 mm of the superior continuation of a line drawn along the posterior cortex of the body of the axis, and the distance of the basion and tip of the odontoid is normally < 12 mm.

467.C. There are many more sodium channels located at the axon hillock. Synaptic inputs are summated in the region of the action hillock and the action potential is initiated here.

468.B. Ganglioglioma is twice as common as dysembryoplastic neuroepithelial tumors (DNET) in causing temporal lobe epilepsy. Gangliogliomas occur mostly in children and young adults, and calcification is frequently present on imaging studies of these tumors.

469.E. Huntington's chorea is not an indication for radiosurgery.

470.E. There is a tendency for the posterior insula to drain more frequently into the deep system, whereas the anterior portion of the insula drains to the superficial venous system.

471.D. The primary fissure separates the anterior cerebellar lobe from the posterior cerebellar lobe. The horizontal fissure is located within the posterior lobe. The dorsolateral fissure is synonymous with the posterolateral fissure and separates the flocculonodular lobe from the posterior lobe.

472.E. Dural arteriovenous (AV) fistulas have a male predominance, are acquired lesions, have low flow, rarely hemorrhage, and have a gradual onset of symptoms.

473.B. Neurons in the penumbra (8–23 mL/100 g/min) survive but do not function. Below 8 mL/100 g/min neurons cannot recover. Hypothermia can allow a modestly prolonged survival at these blood flows.

474.C. The zona incerta is the gray matter between the thalamic and lenticular fasciculi. Laterally, the zona incerta is continuous with the thalamic reticular nucleus.

475.D. Evidence for these areas influencing micturition comes from positron emission tomographic scanning.

476.C. The juxtarestiform body carries both afferent and efferent fibers connecting the vestibular nuclei and the flocculonodular lobe and fastigial nucleus of the cerebellum. It coordinates balance and eye movements by communication between the vestibular apparatus and the cerebellum.

477.C. Type II fibers connect to nuclear chain fibers and static nuclear bag fibers. These connections are flower-spray endings and insert into the ends of the fiber.

478.B. In a caudalis dorsal root entry zone (DREZ) operation, the electrode penetrates the dorsal spinocerebellar tract into the trigeminal tract and deeper caudalis nucleus.

479.C. The arterial dicrotic notch corresponds to the area between the tidal (P2) and dicrotic (P3) peaks of the ICP waveform.

480.A. The basal vein of Rosenthal receives tributaries from the medial temporal lobe and brainstem. It begins at the anterior perforated substance.

481.C.   The trigone of the lateral ventricle is a triangular area defined by the temporal horn inferiorly, the occipital horn posteriorly, and the body of the lateral ventricle anteriorly.

482.D.   Decussation of the superior cerebellar peduncles occurs in the caudal midbrain tegmentum at the level of the inferior colliculus. The superior cerebellar peduncle is one of the structures that connects the cerebellum to the midbrain. The ventral spinocerebellar tract enters the cerebellum through the superior cerebellar peduncle.

483.B.   The ascending pharyngeal artery supplies these nerves before anastomosing with vertebral artery branches. This artery also supplies the pharynx.

484.B.   Destruction of the abducens nucleus (subcortical center for lateral gaze) results in an ipsilateral lateral rectus and contralateral medial rectus palsy on attempted lateral gaze.

485.B.   Brainstem auditory evoked responses test the ear and the brain. They measure the timing of electrical waves from the brainstem in response to clicks in the ear. Waveforms represent specific anatomical points along the auditory pathway.

486.D.   The lateral subnucleus of CN III innervates the inferior rectus, inferior oblique, and medial rectus. The medial subnucleus innervates the contralateral superior rectus. The central subnucleus innervates the levator palpebrae superioris.

487.C.   The primary sensory cortex is Brodmann areas 3, 1, and 2. This area of the cortex is organized somatotopically, having the pattern of a homunculus.

488.B.   Pain is more common in cauda equina lesions than in conus lesions. Motor loss is more marked in cauda lesions, and bladder and rectum are involved later in cauda lesions. The onset of cauda lesions is more gradual than that of conus lesions. Also cauda lesions are more commonly unilateral than conus lesions. Cauda equina lesions can occur with compression in the lower lumbar region, they are a medical emergency, and patients should be admitted with urgent surgery to decompress the nerves and stabilize the spine if necessary. Approximately 1% of a busy spine practice can be cauda equina conditions, yet insurance companies and some hospitals will incorrectly and unethically insist that such surgeries can be performed electively at a later time for cost savings.

489.C.   MPNSTs are also known as schwannomas, neurofibrosarcomas, and neuro-sarcomas. The trigeminal nerve is most commonly involved only because it is the largest cranial nerve.

490.D.   The superior ophthalmic vein courses into the anterior cavernous sinus above the sixth nerve and below the first division of the trigeminal nerve. The superior ophthalmic vein is exterior to the annulus of Zinn.

491.E.   The caudate nucleus forms the lateral wall of the frontal horn, body, and trigone of the lateral ventricle. It forms the roof of the temporal horn. The caudate does not extend to the occipital horn. The caudate nucleus makes up the basal ganglia along with the putamen and globus pallidus.

492.E.   The dorsal trigeminothalamic tract is the rostral equivalent of the dorsal-column medial-lemniscal system.

493.D.   The loose areolar tissue contains the valveless emissary veins. Emissary veins connect the extracranial venous system with the intracranial venous sinuses.

494.A.   Apocrine sweat glands of the axilla are innervated by adrenergic fibers and secrete in response to mental stress. The eccrine sweat glands have cholinergic innervation.

495.B.   The water content of the nucleus pulposus is maximum at birth and declines throughout life, the greatest decline occurring during the growth phase in childhood.

496.C.   The tapetum are corpus callosum fibers connecting the temporal and occipital lobes.

497.D.   Apraxia is a disorder of motor planning. Dressing apraxia can be tested by having the patient put on a jacket with the sleeves first deliberately turned inside-out.

498.C.   Cerebrospinal fluid is reabsorbed into the bloodstream through pressure-sensitive one-way valves in the arachnoid villi.

499.D.   Proopiomelanocortin (POMC) gives rise to adrenocorticotropic hormone (ACTH) and beta-lipotropin. ACTH gives rise to alpha-MSH and CLIP. Beta-lipotropin gives rise to beta-endorphin and gamma-lipotropin.

500.E.   Late-onset myasthenia gravis (onset after age 50) is more common in males. Early-onset myasthenia gravis (onset from ages 18 to 50) is more common in females.

501.D.   The ICA enters the cranium via the carotid canal of the temporal bone.

502.E.   Damage to the trochlear nucleus results in damage to the contralateral superior oblique because the fibers decussate in the superior medullary velum.

503.A.   The asterion is located at the intersection of the lambdoid, occipitomastoid, and parietomastoid sutures. This point reliably marks the anteroposterior level of the transverse-sigmoid sinus junction.

504.D.   The anterior nucleus of the hypothalamus is involved in thermal regulation (dissipation of heat). The anterior nucleus stimulates the parasympathetic nervous system. Destruction of this nucleus results in hyperthermia.

505.D.   Disks make up roughly 25% of the spine's height. There is no disk at the occipitoatlantal joint, atlantoaxial joint, sacrum, or coccyx. Traction and inversion table therapy can help to slow down the desiccation and shortening of disk space height.

506.C.   SIADH is a type of hyponatremia characterized by euvolemia.

507.D.   Duane's syndrome produces a characteristic pattern of eye movement with failure of abduction and retraction of the globe on adduction; the third nerve innervates the lateral rectus due to developmental failure of motor neurons in the sixth nerve nucleus. Alexander Duane was an American ophthalmologist who published "A New Classification of the Motor Anomalies of the Eye" in 1897.

508.C.   Dilantin levels are decreased by carbamazepine.

509.A.   Olivocerebellar fibers end as climbing fibers, and aspartate is a common neurotransmitter in this connection. Reticulocerebellar and pontocerebellar fibers end as mossy fibers.

510.A.   Paraganglioma is a rare neuroendocrine neoplasm the great majority of which are benign. About 3% of these tumors are malignant and are able to produce distant metastases. Tumor location is often more relevant than histology and other factors in assessing the prognosis of paraganglioma patients. For example, the metastatic rate of para-aortic paraganglioma is high (~ 30%), whereas that of carotid body tumors is much lower (~ 6%). Most paragangliomas are either asymptomatic or present as a painless mass.

511.C.   The anteromedial triangle of the middle fossa can be used to expose portions of the cavernous sinus and lateral sphenoid wing.

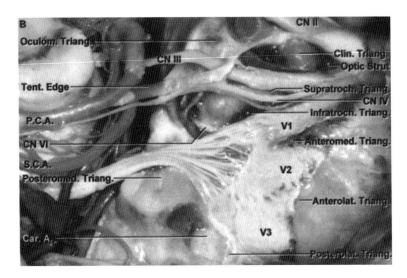

512.B.   Hyperperfusion encephalopathy is believed to result from the failure of intracranial vessels to compensate adequately for rapid increases of blood pressure. The posterior brain regions exhibit reversible edema bilaterally. This condition is also known as PRES (posterior reversible encephalopathy syndrome). Patients can present with headaches, seizures, and/or visual disturbances.

513.A.   Glasscock's triangle is also known as the posterolateral triangle. Its contents are the foramen spinosum, horizontal petrous ICA, and infratemporal fossa.

514.C.   The posterior circulation has sparse sympathetic innervation and is less well protected from hyperperfusion encephalopathies.

515.D.   The central sulcus rarely joins the lateral sulcus. The central sulcus separates the parietal lobe from the frontal lobe and the primary motor cortex from the primary sensory cortex. This was originally called the fissure of Rolando after Luigi Rolando, an Italian anatomist who published extensively on brain anatomy and function in the 1800s.

516.B.   Ipsilateral flushing is seen with cluster headaches. Cluster headaches also have an increased intraocular pressure, increased local skin temperature, and male predominance, and are seen in older patients. Migraine headaches can be improved with Botox (Allergan) injections to the scalp musculature. Many patients given the diagnosis of migraine headaches may have cervicogenic headaches, and a cervical MRI is helpful in determining this. Cervicogenic headaches have a characteristic triad of headache, pressure behind the eye, and a swooshing sound (or tinnitus) in the ear.

517.E. The syndrome described is Balint's syndrome. It is of interest to note that functional "streams" of visual processing have been postulated. The "where" stream is destined for further processing in the parietal lobes and subserves spatial localization and the control of eye movements. The "what" stream is destined for the temporal lobes and is concerned with the identification of objects and color vision. Evidence for this came from studying patients with Balint's syndrome.

518.D. The amygdala is not removed completely in this procedure. The most medial part abuts the basal ganglia, anterior commissure, and tail of the caudate.

519.A. The anterior choroidal artery can be divided into two segments: the cisternal segment extends from its origin until the choroidal fissure and the intraventricular segment after entering the choroidal fissure.

520.D. The gluteus minimus is a medial rotator of the thigh. The others listed are all lateral rotators. The gluteus minimus is the smallest of the three gluteal muscles. Paralysis of this muscle may be caused by a superior gluteal nerve palsy.

521.C. Lewy bodies are concentrically laminated, round bodies found in vacuoles in the cytoplasm. They are absent in multiple system atrophy (MSA). Lewy bodies were discovered by Frederic Lewy, an American neurologist.

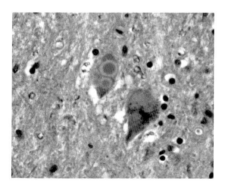

522.B. The thalamostriate vein lies in the groove between the thalamus and caudate nucleus and receives blood from both.

523.B. Paresthesias of the fingertips or mouth indicate that the electrode is too posterior (in the region of the ventralis caudalis [VC]). The electrode needs to be repositioned more anteriorly. High-frequency stimulation of the VC causes contralateral paresthesias. The threshold for inducing contralateral paresthesias is higher in the ventralis intermedius (Vim) (target), and it is usually > 3 V.

524.C.   Deficiency of the late complement components predisposes to *Neisseria meningitidis*. Deficiency of early complement components tend to be linked with autoimmune diseases. Complement deficiencies are said to comprise between 1 and 10% of all primary immunodeficiencies.

525.B.   Meningiomas and choroid plexus papillomas are the most common neoplasms of the trigone of the lateral ventricle. Meningiomas originate from the arachnoid cap cells of the choroid plexus and the tela choroidea. Intraventricular meningiomas present in mid adulthood with a female predilection.

526.B.   The status of systemic disease is the most important determinant for survival.

527.B.   Golgi tendon organs are associated with Ib (A-a) fibers. Muscle spindles are associated with Ia (A-a) fibers. Slow pain and temperature are carried by unmyelinated fibers IV (C).

528.C.   *Staphylococcus aureus* causes ~ 60–90% of cases of spinal epidural abscesses. The most frequent location is the thoracic epidural space.

529.D.   There is a greater risk of shunt infection with proximal revisions.

530.B.   The development of sarcomas after cranial irradiation is well described. Fibrosarcomas are the most common type arising in the sella after irradiation for pituitary tumors.

531.D.   Dopamine plays a central role in Parkinson's disease, attention deficit hyperactivity disorder, schizophrenia, and drug addiction.

532.D.   The sequence of antidiuretic hormone (ADH) release after surgery is triphasic. Initially, excessive diuresis is due to disruption of the pituitary stalk. Then there is a release of ADH in large amounts from degeneration of distal axons. Finally the stored ADH disappears, and excessive diuresis returns.

533.E.   Patients with infection commonly present with cord compression due to the predilection of echinococcus for bone, particularly vertebrae. Within bone tissue hyatid cysts enlarge by daughter cyst formation. The goal of surgery is removal of the cysts; an anterior or circumferential approach is recommended.

534.B. The mediodorsal nucleus is reciprocally connected to the prefrontal cortex. The prefrontal cortex is the cerebral cortex, which covers the front part of the frontal lobe. It contains Brodmann areas 9, 10, 11, 12, 46, and 47.

535.C. Lymphoma metastatic to the brain tends to localize to the meninges, as opposed to the intraparenchymal (often subependymal) location of primary tumors.

536.C. The hippocampal commissure is located in the posterior component of the forniceal structure.

537.E. The centromedian nucleus is reciprocally connected to the motor cortex (area 4).

538.B. During surgery around the mastoid process, care must be taken to avoid injury to cranial nerve VII as it exits through the stylomastoid foramen, which is located medial to the insertion of the posterior belly of the digastric muscle at the digrastric groove.

539.D. In addition, postoperative amnesia may result from manipulation of the fornix.

540.D. The rostral one-third of the red nucleus receives dentate fibers, and the caudal two-thirds receive fibers from the interposed nuclei. Stimulation of the red nucleus elicits increased tone in the contralateral flexors. The red nucleus gets its pale pink color from hemoglobin and ferritin, which are present in the red nucleus.

541.E. Phenoxybenzamine is a nonselective, irreversible alpha blocker used in the treatment of hypertension, especially hypertension caused by pheochromocytoma. It is also used in complex regional pain syndrome type 1 due to its antiadrenergic effects.

542.E. Ketamine anesthesia increases $CMRO_2$. All other anesthetic drugs decrease $CMRO_2$. The main energy demands of the brain are those of ion flux related to excitation and conduction. Continuous cerebral circulation is absolutely required to provide sufficient oxygen.

543.D. The globus pallidus projects to three thalamic nuclei via the thalamic fasciculus (FFH1).

544.D.   The major blood supply to ventricular trigone meningiomas is constant, arising from the anterior choroidal artery, with only a minor component arising from the posterior choroidal artery.

545.D.   Elevated markers are indicative of malignant germ cell tumors, and these tumors can be radiosensitive and chemosensitive, precluding surgery.

546.A.   The crus cerebri is the anterior portion of the cerebral peduncle, which contains motor tracts.

547.C.   The Glasgow Coma Scale (GCS) score is 9. She opens eyes to pain (2) and mumbles sounds (2), and the best motor response is localizing (5). Always take the best motor response when assessing GCS. An intracerebral pressure monitor may not be indicated with a patient who is localizing. The CT brain and neuro exam can guide treatment in this particular patient.

548.B.   (Or C.) Ewing's sarcoma may present with involvement of the dura, skull, and possibly the underlying parenchyma.

549.E.   This is a calvarial metastases, an occurrence observed not uncommonly with metastatic breast carcinoma.

550.D.   Sinunasal carcinoma may metastasize to multiple dural-based locations.

551.B.   Recurrence after maximal radiation is an indication to operate.

552.B.

553.C.   Diphtheria toxin has a predilection to sensory and motor nerves of the limbs and ciliary muscles or nerves.

554.A.   Tetanus may typically present with trismus, risus sardonicus, tonic spasms, and generalized convulsions.

555.B.   Symptoms appear 12–48 hours after ingestion and may be preceded by nausea, vomiting, and diarrhea. The convergence difficulty is usually followed by ptosis and extraocular muscle paralysis.

556.D.   This is a typical feature of Reye's syndrome.

557.C.   Patients with spinal multiple myeloma typically present with hypercalcemia, bone pain characteristically absent at rest, and spinal canal invasion in about 10% of cases. Multiple myeloma (MM) and amyloid light-chain (AL) amyloidosis are caused by the expansion of monoclonal plasma cells and secretion of dysproteinemia (Bence Jones protein and free light chain).

558.B.   Myeloma cells in two or more peripheral blood smears are required.

559.C.   It represents spread via spinal epidural veins. The Batson venous plexus is a network of valveless veins in the human body that connect the deep pelvic veins and thoracic veins to the internal vertebral venous plexuses.

560.C.   Facioscapulohumoral dystrophy, or Landouzy-Dejerine's syndrome is associated with a defect on chromosome 4.

561.A.   Werdnig-Hoffmann's disease has autosomal recessive inheritance on chromosome 5q.

562.E.   Myotonic muscular dystrophy has autosomal dominant inheritance on chromosome 19.

563.B.   Cri du chat syndrome is due to a 5p deletion and results in microcephaly, hypertelorism, and congenital heart disease.

564.D.   Friedreich's ataxia has autosomal recessive inheritance on chromosome 9. It is named after German pathologist and neurologist Nikolaus Friedreich who identified this disease in 1863.

565.B.   Diltiazem is the preferred agent for patients with systolic heart failure because it produces less myocardial depression than verapamil.

566.A.   Verapamil's side effects include hypotension and worsening of systolic heart failure due to negative inotropic effect.

567.C.   Digoxin is indicated for chronic rate control of atrial fibrillation. Because of its delayed action it is not indicated in acute atrial fibrillation.

568.D. Procainamide is contraindicated in patients with prolonged QT interval because it prolongs QT interval and may be pro-arrhythmic. It is used to convert atrial fibrillation to normal sinus rhythm.

569.E. Beta-blockers are indicated for rate control of atrial fibrillation in the setting of a hyperadrenergic state such as acute myocardial infarction after bypass surgery.

570.B. Gliosarcoma has the same histological features as glioblastoma multiforme. In addition, it does stain for reticulin in the sarcomatous part of the tumor. Approximately 2% of glioblastomas are gliosarcomas.

571.D. Blunt trauma injuries to the cervical vertebral artery are more often managed by ligation than repair. Ligation may be risky since only ~ 20% of the general population has a complete collateral circulation. Proximal occlusion may be accomplished by an anterior approach with mobilization of the sternocleidomastoid. Endovascular treatment with detachable balloons is a valid option for management.

572.C. Arsenic causes peripheral neuropathy, nausea, and vomiting.

573.E. Lead causes encephalitis in children as well as pica, irritability, seizures, abdominal cramping, ataxia, coma, and high intracranial pressure.

574.B. Manganese causes a Parkinson-like syndrome.

575.E.

576.A. Mercury causes peripheral neuropathy, cerebellar signs, psychological dysfunctions, tremor, movement disorders, and renal tubular necrosis.

577.D. Aluminum may present with a picture of Alzheimer's disease.

578.A. Left atrium accounts for 65–75% of embolisms, mainly the left appendage. The left ventricle and ventricular aneurysms account for 5% each.

579.E. Uremia is most likely to cause potassium stores depletion.

580.B. Tetany is the first sign of magnesium depletion. Delirium occurs usually before convulsions. An increase in deep tendon reflexes is usually observed.

581.D. Ca^{2+} concentration is 3 mEq/L.

582.B. The MRI scan demonstrates an intramedullary astrocytoma, which occurs most commonly in the cervical spine. Lower motor signs may be at the level of the lesion and may aid in localization. These types of tumors are the most common intramedullary tumors in children and are usually of fibrillary type. Intramedullary tumors may be treated empirically with cyberknife radiosurgery with good results forgoing the need for biopsy which can be risky. A lumbar puncture may be used for an indirect biopsy which is reasonably safe. It is however low yield but worth a try.

583.C.

584.A.

585.D.

586.C. Rickets disease presents with increased alkaline phosphatase and decreased serum calcium and phosphate levels.

587.D. Paget's disease usually presents with increased alkaline phosphatase and normal serum calcium and phosphate levels; serum calcium levels may be increased depending on the stage of the disease.

588.A. Hyperparathyroidism usually presents with increased alkaline phosphatase, increased serum calcium, and decreased or normal phosphate levels.

589.D. Primary osteoporosis usually presents with increased alkaline phosphatase and normal serum calcium and phosphate levels.

590.B. Hypoparathyroidism usually presents with normal alkaline phosphatase, decreased serum calcium, and increased phosphate levels.

591.E.

592.B.

593.C.

594.A.

595.D. Here are some pointers in interpreting the arterial blood gas: The most useful information comes from the clinical description of the patient by the history and physical examination; however in this case this information is not given. Therefore, the next step is to look at the pH. If pH < 7.35, then there is an acidemia; if pH > 7.45, then there is an alkalemia. The pH may be normal in the presence of a mixed acid base disorder, particularly if other parameters of the ABG are abnormal. The third step is to look at PCO_2 and HCO_{3-} in order to determine the acid base process (alkalosis vs. acidosis) leading to the abnormal pH. In simple acid base disorders, both values are abnormal and direction of the abnormal change is the same for both parameters. One abnormal value will be the initial change and the other will be the compensatory response. Once the initial change is identified, then the other abnormal parameter is the compensatory response if the direction of the change is the same. If not, suspect a mixed disorder. Once the initial chemical change and the compensatory response is distinguished, then identify the specific disorder. If PCO_2 is the initial chemical change, then the process is respiratory; if HCO_{3-} is the initial change, then the process is metabolic.

Below is a brief description of the initial chemical change followed by the compensatory response in basic acid/base disorders:

Respiratory Acidosis

↑PCO_2

↑HCO_{3-}

Respiratory Alkalosis

↓PCO_2

↓HCO_{3-}

Metabolic Acidosis

↓HCO_{3-}

↓PCO_2

Metabolic Alkalosis

↑HCO_{3-}

↑PCO_2

596.C.

597.B.

598.A.   Scan 1 shows a wedge infarct and scan 2 shows a watershed infarct, which can also be due to small embolic infarcts. Both endocarditis and occlusive disease of a single artery may result in scan deficits 1. Watershed infarcts may typically present with man-in-the-barrel syndrome due to hypoperfusion. Man-in-the-barrel syndrome is manifested by bilateral arm weakness, intact cranial nerves, and preservation of leg function, appearing as if the upper limbs were confined in a barrel. It is most frequently caused by cerebral vascular disorders and cardiac surgeries involving arterial hypotension, and the spinal cord may be involved as well. Other cases of man-in-the-barrel syndrome may be due to cerebral metastases, hemorrhagic contusion in trauma, ALS, and lower motor neuron disease.

599.B.   The preoptic nucleus is considered part of the anterior hypothalamus.

600.C.   All the other choices result in an efferent defect.

601.D.   Metabolic neuropathy is typically symmetric and bilateral and will rarely present with an afferent pupillary defect clinically.

602.C.   An improvement in mixed venous oxygen contents will often improve the hypoxemia in the setting of a shunt.

603.B.   The half-life is 72 hours.

604.A.   Conversion of prothrombin from thrombin is the most time consuming and is usually measured as the prothrombin time (PT); it is in the range of 11 to 13 seconds.

605.B.   The second figure shows a venous angioma which can be caused by arrested development.

606.D.   Dural arteriovenous malformations are usually acquired after dural thrombosis. Neither cavernous malformation (first image) nor venous angioma (second image) is an acquired lesion.

607.B.   Blue rubber nevus syndrome is associated with venous angiomas.

608.D.

609.C.

610.E.

611.B.

612.A.

613.B.   The glomerulus is formed by the Golgi cell, the granule cell, and the mossy fiber.

614.A.   The granule cell is the only excitatory cell within the cerebellum.

615.D.   Basket cells end in a rete of terminals around the Purkinje cell.

616.C.   Purkinje cells synapse with the deep cerebellar nuclei.

617.D.   Early signs of cyanide poisoning include general weakness, malaise, early giddiness, inebriation, confusion, headache, vertigo, dizziness, confusion, and hallucinations. Tachypnea and hyperpnea generally precede apnea.

618.E.   All are important in wound healing. Zinc is a mineral that is important for the action of collagenase. Manganese is necessary for the glycosylation of hydroxyproline residues in the formation of collagen. Copper is a cofactor of ceruloplasmin and is involved in the synthesis of oxidative metalloenzymes and elastics. Iron is a vital cofactor for proteins and enzymes involved in energy metabolism, respiration, DNA synthesis, cell cycle arrest, and apoptosis.

619.D.   Aminoglycosides act by inhibiting protein synthesis through irreversible ribosomal attachment. Examples of aminoglycoside antibiotics are amikacin, tobramycin, gentamicin, streptomycin, and neomycin.

620.D.   Polymyxin does not cause neuromuscular blockade.

621.B.   The image represents a vertebral artery aneurysm. The preferred treatment is direct aneurysm clipping of this aneurysm. The Allcock test will test patency of the circle of Willis via carotid occlusion. Vasospasm in this area can cause midbrain and medullary syndrome, including respiratory arrest and neurogenic pulmonary edema. A lumbar arachnoid catheter may also be used to allow CSF drainage.

622.B.   When removing an intramedullary spinal cord tumor one is more likely to encounter dilated veins at the caudal end of the mass. The other points are general principles of spinal cord tumor resection. Note that it is useful to seek out the blood supply of the tumor before debulking to keep the field relatively free of blood.

623.A.   Galactocerebroside accumulates in Krabbe's disease. Ganglioside accumulates in Tay–Sachs's and Sandhoff's diseases. Long chain fatty acids accumulate in adrenoleukodystrophy.

624.C.   The T-reflex represents the monosynaptic stretch reflex elicited by tapping a tendon.

625.C.   The trochlear nerve arises at the level of the lower midbrain (inferior colliculus level).

626.D.   The patient likely has Lambert–Eaton myasthenic syndrome (LEMS) with small cell (oat cell) carcinoma. About 60% of those with LEMS have an underlying malignancy, most commonly small cell lung cancer.

627.B.   Total body potassium excess of 100 to 200 mEq is required to produce a rise of 1 mEq/L in serum potassium.

628.B.   The ulnar nerve has no supply from the C6 root.

629.B.   Cervical roots C2 and C3 innervate this muscle.

630.D.   Involved in the phrenic nerve and the brachial plexus.

631.C.   Innervated by the obturator nerve (L2, L3).

632.D.   Innervated by C3, C4 (cervical nerves) and C5 (dorsal scapular nerve which arises from the brachial plexus).

633.E.   Innervated by the pudendal nerve (S2–S4).

634.B.   Innervated by the accessory nerve and C2 roots.

635.A.   Hypnagogic hallucinations are seen with narcolepsy. Hypnagogic or hypno-pompic hallucinations are visual, tactile, auditory, or other sensory events, usually brief but occasionally prolonged, that occur at the transition from wakefulness to sleep (hypnagogic) or from sleep to wakefulness (hypnopo-mpic). People with narcolepsy have a reduced number of neurons that pro-duce the protein orexin-A.

636.E.   Vitamin A intoxication is associated with pseudotumor cerebri.

637.A.   Beriberi is associated with thiamin deficiency (B1). Beriberi is divided into three separate entities depending on which body system is involved: periph-eral nervous system (dry beriberi), cardiovascular system (wet beriberi), or gastrointestinal system.

638.C.   Increased serum homocysteine and methylmalonic acid is associated with vitamin B12 deficiency.

639.B.   Pyridoxine deficiency is associated with lower extremity paresthesias.

640.A.   Barbiturates are used as antiepileptics and in the treatment of intractable increased intracranial pressure.

641.C.   Both picrotoxin and bicuculline are GABA receptor blockers.

642.B.   Baclofen in used as a centrally acting muscle relaxant. Baclofen can be ad-ministered transdermally, orally, or intrathecally.

643.C.   Bicuculline is a selective GABA-A antagonist directly at the site where GABA binds.

644.E.   The two aneurysms are a calcified thrombotic basilar artery aneurysm and a posterior communicating artery aneurysm.

645.D.   The lesion presented is a colloid cyst of the third ventricle. A lumbar punc-ture is contraindicated prior to the placement of a shunt or a ventricular catheter due to the risk of herniation.

646.D.   Torsades de pointes presents with prolonged QT intervals.

647.C.   In early ARDS, the chest X-ray may be unrevealing, whereas the patient may present with a hypoxemia refractory to supplemental oxygen.

648.B. Bicarbonate therapy does not improve outcome in diabetic ketoacidosis, regardless of the severity of the acidosis.

649.B. The MRI shows an enhancing mural nodule with an associated cyst. Pathology shows highly vascular tissue and stromal cells characteristic of hemangioblastoma.

650.D. This T2-weighted MRI shows enhancement of the medial temporal lobe, a finding representative of herpes encephalitis.

651.B. The superficial peroneal nerve innervates the peroneus longus and brevis, which evert the foot. A lesion of the deep peroneal nerve will affect ankle dorsiflexion. A lesion of the common peroneal or sciatic nerves will affect both ankle dorsiflexion and foot eversion. A sciatic nerve lesion will also affect foot flexion and inversion.

652.C. The order of the brachial plexus structures is: root, trunk, division, cord, and branch.

653.C. Fissure splitting, temporary clipping, dissection of M2 branch from dome, and definitive clipping is the proper order of steps for clipping this difficult aneurysm.

654.D. Aberrations of genes coding for cell cycle regulatory proteins involved in the control of G_1/S phase transition have been found in gliomas and include mutation or deletion of genes like p53, retinoblastoma, cyclic AMP-dependent kinase number 2 (CDKN2) A/B, and amplification or overexpression of CDK4 and CDK6.

655.B. Oligodendrogliomas may exhibit loss of chromosomal regions on 1p and 19q13. Other chromosomal regions that may be lost from oligodendrogliomas are 1p36, 9p, and 22. There may be evidence of increased numbers of chromosome 7.

656.D. The superior hypogastric plexus lies in front of the promontory of the sacrum between the two common iliac arteries and is sometimes called the presacral nerve. It then divides into the right and left inferior hypogastric plexuses.

657.C.

658.C.

659.B.   The circuit of Papez includes the cingulate gyrus, hippocampus, mammillary bodies, and anterior nucleus of the thalamus. The lateral parabrachial nucleus of the amygdala receives inputs from the lateral olfactory tract, pyriform cortex, hypothalamus, paraventricular thalamus, and solitary tract nucleus. The medial septal nucleus projects to the fimbria to the hippocampus.

660.D.   AIDS is frequently associated with platelet disorders.

661.D.   This MRI scan shows a vein of Galen malformation, which is usually associated with macrocephaly and hydrocephalus.

662.A.   The following MRI scan demonstrates an epidural abscess, which more frequently occur in the thoracolumbar region.

663.B.   Urinary magnesium loss is most prominent with loop diuretics.

664.C.   The superior salivatory nucleus sends axons via the nervus intermedius (VII) to the greater superficial petrosal nerve and then to the pterygopalatine ganglion.

665.D.   The oculomotor nerve (III) carries parasympathetics from Edinger–Westphal's nucleus to the ciliary ganglion.

666.A.   Arnold's nerve is a branch of the vagus nerve (X) supplying sensation to the dura of the posterior fossa.

667.E.   The deep petrosal nerve carries sympathetic fibers from the internal carotid artery from the superior cervical ganglion.

668.A.   Both nerves contain sensory inputs from the outer ear. The glossopharyngeal nerve controls elevation of the pharynx, whereas the facial nerve has no actions on pharyngeal muscles.

669.B.   Dobutamine is an adrenergic agent that does not cause peripheral vasoconstriction.

670.B.   Thiocyanate is cleared by the kidneys and its accumulation with the use of nitroprusside may cause a toxic syndrome.

671.B.   Single punched out lesion without sclerotic edges is typical.

672.B. Eosinophilic granuloma may be a monostotic form of Langerhans cell histiocytosis.

673.C. In Paget's disease, one may observe bony destruction (early) and sclerosis (late).

674.A. Albright's syndrome is characterized by unilateral fibrous dysplasia, pigmented skin lesions, and precocious puberty.

675.D. Epidermoid has characteristic scalloped edges.

676.A. *Pneumocystis carinii* pneumonia is the most common cause of ICU admission in HIV-positive patients. It is usually treated with trimethoprim-sulfamethoxazole. Toxoplasma is the most common intracranial infection in HIV-positive patients.

677.C. There are 9 cases of transmission for every 10,000 exposures. It is advisable to wear two pairs of gloves at surgery and to replace the top pair every 90 minutes of arduous surgery.

678.D. The lesion most likely represents a lobulated arachnoid cyst. An aneurysm would not display such septations.

679.D.

680.A. The Golgi organelle possesses enzymes that are important in sugar and lipid chemistry of the eukaryotic cell.

681.B. The endoplasmic reticulum is important in drug detoxification; for example, adding hydroxyl groups to a lipid soluble–type compound makes it more water soluble and thus easier to remove from the body.

682.B. Glycogen formation and breakdown occur in the endoplasmic reticulum; this is particularly important in the liver. Glycogen, a polymer of glucose-1-phosphate, represents a quick source of energy.

683.C. Both the Golgi membranes closest to the nucleus (forming face) and the endoplasmic reticulum have a lamellar or tube-like membranous system. The Golgi membranes away from the nucleus (maturing face) are much more like plasma or organelle membranes.

684.C.   True melanin is made by tyrosinase. Tyrosinase is an oxidase that is the rate-limiting enzyme for controlling the production of melanin. Neuromelanin is biosynthesized from L-dopa by tyrosine hydroxylase and aromatic acid decarboxylase.

685.A.   The amygdala sends efferents to the nucleus accumbens via the amygdalostriate fibers. All others are afferent sources to the amygdala.

686.D.   Total parenteral nutrition has been known to cause hypercapnia due to excessive carbohydrates promoting carbon dioxide retention, impaired oxygenation due to fatty acid damage to pulmonary capillaries, and acalculous cholecystitis due to bile stasis secondary to absence of lipids in the proximal small bowel.

687.A.   This scan shows a teratoma, which is associated with elevation of CEA levels.

688.B.   Paraneoplastic sensory neuropathy with anti-Hu antibodies is associated with limbic encephalitis (as seen on this MRI scan), seizures, epilepsia partialis continua, cerebellar ataxia, autonomic instability, myelitis with patchy weakness, and brainstem encephalitis.

689.A.   Tabes dorsalis presents 15 to 20 years after initial syphilitic infection and is characterized by dorsal root and posterior column involvement as seen on this myelin-stained cord section.

690.C.

691.B.

692.B.

693.A.   Massive pulmonary embolism can result in significant increased dead space and respiratory acidosis; on the other hand, smaller pulmonary embolisms can present with hyperventilation and hence respiratory alkalosis. Liver cirrhosis may also cause hyperventilation. Aminoglycosides can be presynaptic at the neuromuscular junction, causing respiratory acidosis.

694.B.   Tractography is a procedure to demonstrate the neural tracts. It uses special techniques of magnetic resonance imaging (MRI), and computer postprocessing. Information about direction of flow is provided by tractography but not about connections between different structures in the brain.

695.A. The scan shows an atypical dermoid cyst. Dermoid cysts can contain fat which gives them high signal intensity on T1-weighted sequences. A congenital dermal sinus tract can be associated with a dermoid cyst. Choice B is associated with paraganglioma. Choice C is representative of Antoni A pattern in acoustic neuromas.

696.C. The MRI scan shows bilateral acoustic neuromas, pathognomonic of neurofibromatosis type 2. Intertriginous freckling is a feature of neurofibromatosis type 1.

697.D. Carbonic anhydrase inhibitors (e.g., acetazolamide) can cause proximal renal tubular acidosis.

698.C. Methylprednisolone is not recommended in the treatment of emergent Addisonian crisis. Long-term use of methylprednisolone can cause Addisonian crisis if stopped abruptly and not tapered.

699.D. All three medications have been shown to help in the treatment of syndrome of inappropriate antidiuretic hormone (SIADH), with variable side-effect patterns.

700.A. Plasma types B and O can be safely transfused in a patient with blood type B because both of these plasma types do not contain antibodies against B type blood.

701.E. Neurogenic shock is characterized by dilatation of arterioles and venules and decreased peripheral vascular resistance. It also presents with warm, dry skin, bradycardia, and hypotension.

702.A. The urinary system is the most commonly involved in patients with gram-negative septicemia, followed by the respiratory system.

703.C. Stool culture has a sensitivity of > 90% in diagnosing *C. difficile* enterocolitis. Both latex agglutination and tissue culture assay for cytotoxin have a sensitivity of ~ 70%. Stool microscopy is not used to diagnose this condition.

704.D. Halothane increases cerebral blood flow the most followed by enflurane and isofurane.

705.C. Thiopental decreases intracranial pressure. The other listed agents will increase intracranial pressure.

706.A.   Isofurane has been shown to cause tachycardia transiently in children.

707.B.   Enfurane increases systemic vascular resistance. Isofurane will decrease it.

708.C.   Both NF1 and NF2 have autosomal dominant patterns of inheritance.

709.D.   Retinal hemangiomas are associated with von Hippel–Lindau disease.

710.A.   Iris hamartomas or Lisch nodules are seen in NF1.

711.D.   Neurofibromatosis type 5 is the segmental type.

712.E.   The anterior clinoid process is most likely going to have to be drilled to gain access to the neck of this aneurysm.

713.C.   The superior cerebellar artery is seen in neurovascular conflict with the trigeminal nerve. More proximally though, the artery is seen near the tentorium which is in very close relation to the trochlear nerve.

714.A.   The posterior approach is unfavorable in this case since the angle of the tentorium is very steep and would necessitate severe retraction on the cerebellum. In addition, the posterior approach presents a very narrow corridor limited by the internal cerebral veins.

715.D.

716.C.

717.B.

718.C.

719.A.   Papaverine inhibits antiparkinsonian effect of levodopa. Fluconazole increases serum phenytoin and decreases warfarin metabolism. Thyroid hormones enhance clotting factor catabolism. Meperidine may cause hypertension, rigidity, and excitation when used with monoamine oxidase inhibitors.

720.D.   The other medications will tend to further exacerbate the symptoms of malignant hyperthermia.

721.C.   Colon carcinoma has a predilection to metastasize to the liver and other visceral organs.

722.B. The lateral, medial, and posterior cords carry their names in relation to the second and third segments of the axillary artery.

723.C. This type of spondylolisthesis is caused by a defect in the pars interarticularis, occurs in 90% of cases at L5–S1, and is usually bilateral and more common in males.

724.D. The superior outer quadrantanopia is due to involvement of Willebrand's knee.

725.A.

726.A.

727.C.

728.B. Meyer's loops are interrupted causing a homonymous superior quadrantanopia.

729.E.

730.B. Ulnar nerve entrapment can occur at the arcade of Struthers.

731.C. Extensor carpi ulnaris palsy may be due to a constriction at the arcade of Frohse.

732.A. The brachial artery along with the median nerve pass under the Struthers ligament.

733.A. Reservoir sign, or intermittent large volume CSF rhinorrhea, is a relatively uncommon occurrence in patients with sphenoid sinus encephaloceles. The leakage of fluid is usually insidious.

734.B. Scoliosis occurs in 66%, whereas radicular pain occurs in 50% of patients.

735.C. Weakness occurs in 51%, whereas radicular pain occurs in 44% and scoliosis in 36% of patients.

736.D. All are valid mechanisms.

737.D.   De Quervain's syndrome is characterized by tenosynovitis of the abductor pollicis longus and extensor pollicis brevis muscles. The nerve conduction velocities are typically normal.

738.A.

739.B.

740.B.

741.B.   The roof of the fourth ventricle contains both the superior and inferior medullary veli. The floor of the fourth ventricle is formed by the rhomboid fossa, which contains the facial colliculus and hypoglossal trigone.

742.C.   The scan shows a cephalohematoma which is treated with head wrapping and possibly needle aspiration.

743.B.   The notochord induces the formation of the neural plate and neural tube. The neural tube regions give rise to the alar and the basal plates. The alar plate contains sensory/integrative nerve cell bodies of the brain and spinal cord and gives rise to the dorsal horns. The basal plate contains motor neurons of the brain and spinal cord and gives rise to the ventral horn.

744.C.

745.D.

746.B.

747.A.   Cheyne–Stokes respiration occurs with diencephalon lesions. Central neurogenic hyperventilation occurs with midbrain lesions. Apneustic respiration occurs with pontine lesions. Ataxic respiration occurs with medulla lesions.

748.B.

749.A.   The middle cerebellar peduncle contains only afferent fibers.

750.B.   The angiogram demonstrates a primitive trigeminal artery. The persistent acoustic artery passes through the internal auditory meatus.

751.E. The overall rate of HIV transmission from a single percutaneous exposure to HIV-infected blood with high viral load is of the order of 0.3%. Postexposure prophylaxis (PEP) has been shown in one study to reduce this rate by 80%. It is important to check viral loads of patients prior to elective surgery to keep operating room staff and surgeons safe.

752.D. Epidemiological studies of health care workers exposed to hepatitis C virus through a needlestick or other percutaneous injury have found that the incidence of infection averages 1.8% per injury.

753.D. The risk of acquiring hepatitis B from a needlestick when the source was hepatitis B antigen-positive ranges from approximately 2 to 40%, depending on the source's level of viremia.

754.D. The scan shows straight sinus thrombosis.

755.A. Malignant hyperthermia has an autosomal dominant inheritance pattern. It may be caused by halothane or succinylcholine. Body temperature increase is about 1°C every 5 minutes. It is treated with dantrolene and discontinuation of the anesthetic.

756.D. The scan shows a cavernous angioma occurring at the thalamocaudate recess. These lesions may be associated with venous angiomas.

757.A. Type 1 Modic changes show decreased intensity on T1-weighted images and increased intensity on T2-weighted images. Type 2 Modic changes show increased intensity on T1-weighted images and isointense signal intensity on T2-weighted images. Histopathology on type 1 changes demonstrates disruption and fissuring of the end plates and vascularized fibrous tissue. On type 2 changes, yellow marrow replacement is seen. Type 1 changes may convert to type 2 after a few years. There appears to be a spectrum of vertebral body marrow changes associated with degenerative disk disease.

758.D. The lesion represents a syrinx at the level of the inferior cerebellar peduncle. The abducens nerve arises at a higher level and is less likely to be affected. The anterolateral system courses ventral to the lesion and may be affected. The vestibulocochlear nucleus is also located at this level.

759.A. Ketamine raises systemic arterial blood pressure but not necessarily the perfusion in hypovolemic states. In hypotensive states of short duration from endotoxin treatment, it improved the hemodynamics by augmenting the perfusion and the systemic pressure.

760.C.   The scans show a typical intramedullary ependymoma with blockage of CSF flow, which is associated with Froin's syndrome (clotting and xanthochromia in the CSF) and Queckenstedt's sign, which is failure of jugular vein compression to increase CSF. The cervical type of intramedullary ependymoma is usually of the cellular type, more frequent in females in the mid-40s.

761.B.   The MRI set demonstrates basilar meningitis with a trapped fourth ventricle and foramina of Luschka which occurs in sarcoidosis. Elevated angiotensin-converting enzyme levels is also a feature of this disease.

762.B.

763.A.

764.B.

765.C.   The proximal tubule plays a role in secreting organic acids and reabsorbing Na$^+$, water, glucose, bicarbonate, amino acids, and phosphate. The distal tubule's role involves secretion of H$^+$ and K$^+$ and reabsorption of Na$^+$ and Cl. The glomerular filtration rate is at its peak in young adulthood, at about 120 mL/min.

766.A.   The images show craniopharyngioma. The most significant factor associated with recurrence is extent of resection. Histology type is not correlated with frequency of recurrence. MIB-1 LI > 7% is associated with a higher likelihood of recurrence. Malignant transformation to carcinoma exceptionally occurs.

767.A.   Central neurocytoma appears like oligodendroglioma histologically but is positive for synaptophysin on immunohistochemistry.

768.A.   The parietal operculum is caudal to the inferior frontal gyrus. Directly inferior to the inferior frontal gyrus is the sylvian fissure.

769.C.   Nitric oxide promotes the formation of cyclic guanosine monophosphate (cGMP).

770.D.

771.B.

772.C.   Symptomatic 70–90% stenosis of the carotid on angiogram carries a risk of stroke of 26% over 2 years, or 13% per year. Asymptomatic 70–90% stenosis of the carotid on angiogram carries a risk of stroke of 11% over 5 years, or 2% per year. Postcarotid endarterectomy in preoperative symptomatic 70–90% stenosis of the carotid on angiogram carries a risk of stroke of 9% over 2 years, or 4.5% per year.

773.A.   All the other medications cause hyperkalemia.

774.C.   Intracellular methemoglobin appears as hyperintense on T1 and hypointense on T2, and is usually present from 3 days to 2 weeks after a hemorrhage. Extracellular methemoglobin appears after 2 weeks and is hyperintense on T1 and T2. The images show hyperintensity on T1 and iso- to hypointensity on T2, consistent with intracellular methemoglobin toward the end of 2 weeks following the hemorrhage.

775.C.

776.D.   Ethanol has a molecular weight of 46 and is lethal at levels > 350 mg/dL (least lethal). Methanol has the lowest molecular weight (32) and is the least lethal out of the three remaining substances (80 mg/dL needed for lethality). Ethylene glycol has the highest molecular weight (61) and is the most lethal (only 21 mg/dL needed to cause death).

777.E.   Cryoprecipitate is used to treat acute blood loss in von Willebrand's disease.

778.D.   The scan shows a foramen magnum tumor. All the stated clinical findings are associated with this tumor location; however, neurogenic bladder tends to occur very late.

779.D.   Autonomic symptoms occur early.

780.A.   There is no sensory dissociation. Red flags for cauda equina syndrome are erection difficulty, extreme back pain, and groin numbness. An MRI scan taken in a lying down position may not display the stenosis so a standing MRI scan, if available, is necessary. These patients should be sent to an emergency room at once for stat MRI. In the setting of groin numbness only with back pain, urodynamics and Foley catheter may not be absolutely necessary. One should not delay care of these patients to the point in time where urodynamics become necessary. If these patients present in the emergency room, they should not be sent home to follow up electively, they should be decompressed and stabilized on that hospital admission.

	Conus medullaris syndrome	**Cauda equina syndrome**
Presentation	Sudden and bilateral	Gradual and unilateral
Reflexes	Knee jerks preserved but ankle jerks affected	Both ankle and knee jerks affected
Radicular pain	Less severe	More severe
Low back pain	More	Less
Sensory symptoms and signs	Numbness tends to be more localized to perianal area; symmetrical and bilateral; sensory dissociation occurs	Numbness tends to be more localized to saddle area; asymmetrical, may be unilateral; no sensory dissociation; loss of sensation in specific dermatomes in lower extremities with numbness and paresthesia; possible numbness in pubic area, including glans penis or clitoris
Motor strength	Typically symmetric, hyperreflexic distal paresis of lower limbs that is less marked; fasciculations may be present	Asymmetric areflexic paraplegia that is more marked; fasciculations rare; atrophy more common
Impotence	Frequent	Less frequent; erectile dysfunction that includes inability to have erection, inability to maintain erection, lack of sensation in pubic area (including glans penis or clitoris), and inability to ejaculate
Sphincter dysfunction	Urinary retention and atonic anal sphincter cause overflow urinary incontinence and fecal incontinence; tend to present early in course of disease	Urinary retention; tends to present late in course of disease

781.E.   The aorta gives off, from proximal to distal, the brachiocephalic trunk, left common carotid, and left subclavian arteries.

782.B.   With bilateral internuclear ophthalmoplegia there is an adduction deficit in both eyes. This is observed in bilateral lesions of the medial longitudinal fasciculus.

783.A.   Preganglionic sympathetic fibers secrete acetylcholine.

784.B.   The locus ceruleus contains noradrenaline.

785.B.   The periaqueductal gray contains the locus ceruleus. It also contains the dorsal raphe nucleus and enkephalin-releasing neurons.

786.C.   Both Wernicke's and global aphasias display repetition and comprehension deficits.

787.C.   Watershed infarcts occur in areas between the three major vascular territories and are due to a global decrease in cerebral perfusion.

788.D.   McConnell's capsular artery arises directly from the intracavernous carotid artery.

789.D.   Radionuclide scans have a relatively high sensitivity in detecting diskitis.

790.A.   N-acetylaspartate (NAA), found in neurons and axons, is used as a neuronal marker. A reduction in the NAA signal reflects neuronal loss or injury, as seen in many brain pathologies including neurodegenerative diseases. NAA peaks typically represent increased neuronal density. Moderately increased choline peaks and reduced NAA signal intensities indicate low-grade gliomas; high-grade tumors are characterized by distinctly higher choline peaks and even lower NAA signals, and the presence of lipid signals indicates tissue necrosis.

791.B.

792.D.   *Aspergillus* has a predilection for the basal ganglia in some cases. It tends to invade blood vessels, cause hemorrhagic infarcts, and may cause formation of paranasal sinus mycetoma. *Coccidioides* can cause meningitis and caseating granulomas. The diagnosis of early cerebral infarction in a patient considered at risk for invasive aspergillosis, even without overt pulmonary disease, is an indication to institute aggressive antifungal therapy.

793.C.   The MRI scan demonstrates leptomeningeal gliomatosis associated with a high-grade glioma in the left occipital area. The best therapeutic option, given the diffuse nature of the disease is, initially, chemotherapy and radiation.

794.C.   The glossopharyngeal nerve innervates the stylopharyngeus.

795.D.

796.D.

797.B.

798.C.   Functional residual capacity (D) does not change during exercise and is usually 2.4L. It is the sum or residual volume (C) and expiratory reserve volume
(ERV), or the difference between vital capacity (B) and ERV. Vital capacity
(VC) is usually around 4.4 to 5 L and is measured by having the patient in-
hale profoundly and exhale fully into a spirometer. Residual volume cannot
be measured directly and needs to be calculated as a percentage of exhaled
versus inhaled 10% helium-containing solution.

799.C.

800.B.   Point 3 on the MR spectroscopy represents an area of tumor (glioma), which
shows an elevated Chol:Cr ratio and a decreased NAA peak. Other changes
seen in tumors may be decreased Chol and elevated NAA.

801.B.   The formula represents oxygen uptake.

802.D. $(Cc\,O_2 - Ca\,O_2)/(Cc\,O_2 - Cv\,O_2) = Qs/Qt =$ shunt fraction.

803.A. $Q = P\pi r^4/8VL$

804.C.   If the pencil is pulled from his eye, there should be adequate measures to
stop bleeding and irrigate the wound. This can be properly performed only
in the operating room. This patient should be managed with antiepileptic
medication, broad-spectrum antibiotics, CT scan, immediate open surgical
debridement, and follow-up MRI in about a week.

805.D.   The patient has ossification of the posterior longitudinal ligament (OPLL),
which is best managed with cervical corpectomy and fusion. It cannot be
stressed enough that severe cervical compression seen on MRI should be
followed with a CT scan to get an idea of the osteophytes and/or OPLL near
the cord.